A BOOK EVERY DIABETIC MUST READ

HOW TO MANAGE YOUR DIABETES AND LEAD A NORMAL LIFE

A BOOK EVERY DIABETIC MUST READ

HOW TO MANAGE YOUR DIABETES AND LEAD A NORMAL LIFE

Manthappa M.

PEACOCK BOOKS

Published by
PEACOCK BOOKS
B-2, Vishal Enclave, New Delhi-110 027
Phones : 2541 3460, 2542 9987, 2546 6842

Distributed by
ATLANTIC PUBLISHERS AND DISTRIBUTORS (P) Ltd.
7/22, Ansari Road, Darya Ganj, New Delhi-110 002
Phones : 2327 3880, 2327 5880, 2328 0451
Fax : 91-11-2328 5873
E-mail : info@atlanticbooks.com
Web : www.atlanticbooks.com

Branch Office
5, Nallathambi Street, Wallajah Road,
Chennai-600002
Phones : +91-44-64611085, 32413319
e-mail : chennai@atlanticbooks.com

Peacock Books is an imprint of
Atlantic Publishers and Distributors (P) Ltd.

Printed in India at Nice Printing Press, Delhi

Special thanks to

Dr. Raviraj V. Acharya, MD, Professor and Consultant Physician, Kasturba Medical College Hospital, Manipal, for his creative suggestions and foreword.

Mr. M.K. Swamy, my brother, for his encouragement and help while writing this book.

Foreword

It is my pleasure to write a foreword for this innovative book. I know the lives and misery of diabetic patients closely while we interact and treat them in practice. Most of the diabetic patients do not even know the basics of diabetes mellitus. Many diabetics lose their limbs, eyesight and lives due to lack of knowledge about the disease and its poor management. Many people get into a state of shock and depression after learning that they have diabetes or after losing a limb or suffering a stroke. But the simple truth is that every diabetic can lead a completely normal life if he knows what diabetes is and how to manage it. The first step towards managing diabetes is to know as much as possible about it. This knowledge is the one which decides whether a person lives well with diabetes or becomes ill with it. Having diabetes but not knowing about it is like attempting to drive a car without knowing where the brake pedal is. People take an active role in the management of diabetes when they know more about this disease.

India and other developing countries with ever-increasing diabetic population due to multiple factors including change in lifestyle and diet habits need a concerted effort to stall this silent epidemic. Knowledge about the problem in general population is the first step towards this. This will in intermediate and long term reduce the burden of diabetes-related morbidity and mortality. More importantly, this will reduce economic burden on the person, family and society due to prevalence of this disease. Resources, hence, saved can be used for other welfare activities.

The author has made a successful attempt in bringing the medical knowledge to general public in a simple language. I found that every page of this book is packed with vital information and practical tips. One can learn all about diabetes, how to manage it, how to prevent complications, with the help of this book.

I am sure this book will be immensely useful for people with diabetes as also their relatives and care providers. I congratulate the author and my colleague Dr. Manthappa M. for writing this book so lucidly.

Raviraj V. Acharya
MD, DNB (Internal Medicine)
Professor & Senior Consultant Physician
Deputy Executive Editor, *BMJ*, South Asia edition
Kasturba Medical College Hospital, Manipal

Preface

Diabetes is a condition in which blood glucose levels are abnormally high. There are 150 million people with diabetes worldwide, and in India there are more than 30 million people with diabetes. The number of diabetics in India is likely to double in the next 25 years.

Most people get upset when they are told that they have diabetes. If you are diagnosed as diabetic you must be worried and thinking that some incurable disease has happened to you. But cheer up! You are going to be just fine. Diabetes is not a death sentence. Most people with diabetes live long and healthy lives. Nobody dies because of diabetes; people die because of lack of proper management of their diabetes. If diabetes is uncontrolled for a long time, it is likely to damage eyes, kidneys, nerves, and blood vessels. It may also cause infections, sometimes leading to gangrene. Uncontrolled diabetes may lead to heart attack or stroke.

If you are a diabetic patient, just keep cool and put together a practical program to manage your diabetes. You can lead a completely normal life if you know how to manage it. It is fortunate that you know that you have diabetes, because now you are able to take control of your diabetes, prevent complications, and lead a normal life like any other person. There are many people who do not even know that they have diabetes. The first step towards this is that you should know as much as possible about your diabetes because you are the key person in managing your diabetes. The knowledge you have about your diabetes helps you in managing your diabetes more effectively. Your doctor and the rest of your medical team can help you get your diabetes under control but only you can actually do it. In your day-to-day life, you must take care of your diabetes. It is generally accepted that 5 per cent of diabetes care is up to your doctor, and 95% is up to you. So read up! Know as much as you can about diabetes, so that you can deal with it more effectively. This book teaches you all that you need to know about diabetes.

Manthappa M.
MBBS, MD
Consultant Physician
Kasturba Hospital, Manipal

Contents

SOME COMMONLY USED ABBREVIATIONS

DM — Diabetes mellitus.

RBS — Random blood sugar.

FBS — Fasting blood sugar.

PPBS — Postprandial blood sugar.

HbA1c — Hemoglobin A1C.

GRBS, GFBS, GPPBS — These terms mean glucometer RBS, glucometer FBS, and glucometer PPBS. These are nothing but blood sugar tests done by using glucometer.

1 What is Diabetes and Why People get Diabetes?

Diabetes is a condition where blood sugar is high. This high blood sugar may be due to complete absence of insulin in the body (type 1 diabetes) or insufficient insulin in the body or insensitivity of the body to insulin (type 2 diabetes).

Diabetes is not a new disease. Ancient physicians like Charaka (600 BC) and Sushrutha (400 BC) have described all the details of diabetes. They called this disease Madhu-meha (shower of honey). They said that overeating and physical inactivity are the main causes of diabetes.

Why does sugar in the blood become high?

To put it in simple words, this happens because body cannot use sugar. When body cannot use sugar, it accumulates in the blood and becomes high. From where does the sugar come from? Sugar comes from the food that we eat daily. Now let us see in more detail, what happens normally, and what happens in diabetes.

The human body maintains blood glucose (blood sugar) in a very narrow range i.e. between 70–140 mg/dl. When the stomach is empty say in the morning before eating breakfast, blood glucose is usually below 110 mg/dl. After eating food blood glucose starts rising and reaches maximum levels 1-2 hours after eating. This maximum level is usually less than 140 mg/dl. If the blood glucose is above 110 mg/dl on empty stomach or more than 140 mg/dl 2 hours after eating, then you have diabetes mellitus. Blood glucose is maintained within the normal range mainly by two hormones in the blood. These two are insulin and glucagon. Both insulin and glucagon are secreted in an organ called pancreas that lies in the abdomen. Insulin decreases blood sugar by making the body utilize more and

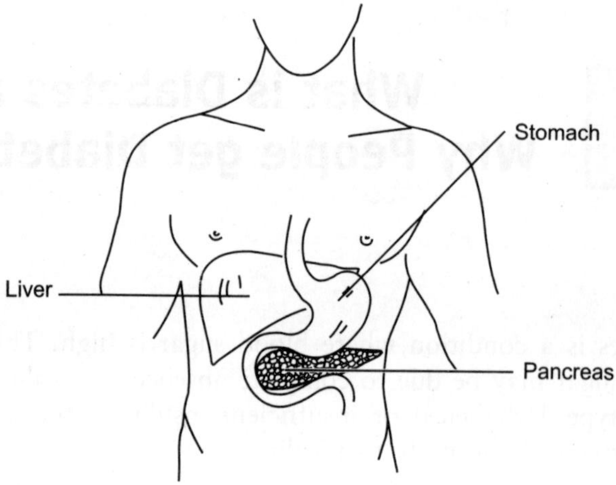

Fig 1.1

more sugar. Glucagon has just the opposite effect. It rises blood sugar by preventing the body from utilizing sugar. The balance between these two hormones maintains biood sugar within the normal range. You may ask why body has two factors with opposite effects on blood sugar. Isn't it enough if we had only insulin. The answer to this question is imagine your car which has an accelerator and a break. One increases the speed and other decreases the speed. And the correct speed is maintained because of both. Similarly, in life we require two opposite things to maintain balance. Glucagon is also as important as insulin. When your blood sugar becomes very low, glucagon is the hormone, which raises blood sugar. There are many situations where blood sugar can become low, for example, while fasting.

Most of the food we eat becomes glucose (sugar) in the body. Glucose is the fuel for the body just like petrol is for car. Glucose is utilized to produce energy required by the body. But, here is a catch. Insulin is required for glucose to be utilized by the body. If there is lack of insulin, glucose cannot be utilized by the body and remains in the blood causing a rise in blood sugar. In simple words, diabetes is nothing but high glucose (sugar) in the blood. So the cause of diabetes is lack of insulin in the body or even if insulin is present in sufficient amounts, it is not able to act.

Lack of insulin in the body has many reasons. Most of the time, it is due to destruction of beta cells of pancreas. Destruction of beta cells of pancreas itself has many reasons. One reason is presence of antibodies reacting against beta cells about which we can do little. Sometimes the pancreas itself may develop some disease like pancreatitis and stop producing insulin.

What makes a person develop diabetes?

Diabetes can occur in anyone and there are many reasons for it. One or more of the following reasons may be responsible for diabetes.

Eating too much food

Eating more than required especially fat and oily food makes you overweight. Once you are overweight, your body starts responding less and less to insulin, which makes your blood sugar to go high. You also develop high BP and high cholesterol because of overweight. It is interesting to note that diabetes is almost unknown in countries where people are poor and cannot afford to overeat.

Being overweight

Also known as obesity, this is the main reason why a person develops diabetes. Because of extra fat in the body be it because of eating more, or doing less work, your body stops responding to insulin, which makes you, develop diabetes.

Always sitting and not doing much physical activity

If you are always sitting and not doing much physical activity, you may develop diabetes. The less active a person is, greater is the risk of developing diabetes. This is because with less physical activity, the body cannot utilize glucose and you become overweight both of which may cause diabetes. Diabetes is uncommon in rural areas where people work hard.

Blood relative has diabetes

Heredity is a major cause of diabetes. A person having a family background of diabetes has 25% more chance of developing diabetes. If both parents have type 2 diabetes, then there is a high chance that their children will develop type 2 diabetes. If both parents have Type 1 diabetes, fewer than 20 per cent of their children will develop Type 1 diabetes. In identical twins, if one twin develops Type 2 diabetes, the chance is nearly 100 per cent that the other twin will also develop it. In Type 1 diabetes, however, there is 40 to 50 per cent chance that second twin will develop the disease.

Age over 40 years

Aging causes many changes in the body. All the organs in our body may not function effectively. That is why old people cannot see and hear properly, have more heart attacks and strokes. Pancreas, which produces insulin, may start producing less insulin, which causes diabetes. However, not all people above 40 years develop diabetes. If you adopt a healthy lifestyle, you may not develop diabetes until you die. On the other hand, even children can develop diabetes because of unhealthy lifestyle.

Enough insulin is there, but the body does not respond to it

Sometimes the body does not respond to insulin, though there is enough insulin in the body. This is known as insulin resistance. This also causes diabetes and is present in type 2 diabetes

Diseases of pancreas

Any illness or disease that damages the pancreas and affects its ability to produce insulin can cause diabetes, e.g. pancreatitis.

Being born in certain races

Hispanics and Americans are at major risk of developing diabetes due to unknown reasons.

Certain medicines

Certain medicines can cause diabetes. E.g. steroids. This type of diabetes is only temporary and goes of after stopping the medicine.

Unknown reasons

In many people, there is no definite cause for diabetes other than the above risk factors. In such persons due to unknown reasons pancreas starts producing lesser insulin than that required by the body and the person becomes diabetic.

Sometimes in a few situations, there may be definite reason for diabetes. If there is a definite reason and if it can be corrected, then the diabetes is curable. However, most of the time there is no such reason and hence diabetes becomes a lifelong disease.

What does not cause diabetes?

Eating sweets and sugar does not cause diabetes

Eating sweets and sugar does not cause diabetes. However, it may make a person overweight, which is a risk factor for developing diabetes. If you are already a diabetic, you need to cut down on sweets to keep your blood sugar under good control.

Excessive stress does not cause diabetes

Stress does not have any direct relation to diabetes. However, if a person already has diabetes stress can make it worse.

Diabetes does not spread from one person to another

Diabetes is not contagious. Someone with diabetes cannot pass it on to anyone else. However, if a close relative has diabetes, then other family members have more chances of developing it. This is not because of close contact but because of genetic predisposition. There may be some genes, which make a person more prone to develop diabetes, and these genes may be transmitted genetically.

Types of diabetes

Diabetes can be classified mainly into 4 types

1. Type 1 diabetes
2. Type 2 diabetes
3. Secondary diabetes
4. Gestational diabetes

Type 1 diabetes

In type 1 diabetes, there is complete absence of insulin in the body. People with type 1 diabetes cannot live without insulin and are dependent on it for their life. Hence, it is also known as insulin dependent diabetes mellitus (IDDM).

Type 2 diabetes

In type 2 diabetes there is some insulin in your body, but it is not adequate for the body. Sometimes there may be normal amount of insulin, but the body may not respond to it normally due to insulin resistance. Type 2 diabetes is the most common type of diabetes and 9 out of 10 cases of diabetes are type 2 diabetes. Type 2 diabetes usually begins after the age of 40 years.

Secondary diabetes

As told earlier, insulin is produced by beta cells of pancreas. If there is damage to pancreas due to some disease like pancreatitis, then insulin production will be less and such a person may develop diabetes.

Gestational diabetes

Gestational diabetes is nothing but diabetes that develops during pregnancy. It is seen only during pregnancy. It goes off after delivery. Hence, doctors test the blood sugar of all the pregnant women when they visit for pregnancy check up because any pregnant woman could be having gestational diabetes.

2 Symptoms of Diabetes

When a person has diabetes, he may have some or all of the following complaints. Note that a diabetic person already on treatment with well-controlled sugars may not have the following complaints.

Passing urine more times

A diabetic person passes large amount of urine more frequently. He has to get up many times at night to pass urine. This happens because, high blood glucose in your body draws water from your tissues, making you feel dehydrated. To quench your thirst, you drink a lot of water and other beverages, which makes you pass large amount of urine more frequently.

Always hungry

Though there is excess sugar in the blood, your body cannot utilize it due to less insulin. Body thinks that there is not enough glucose to supply energy, and makes you eat more. Hence, you feel more hungry than usual.

Feeling thirsty most of the time and in spite of drinking water mouth feels dry

This also happens because high blood glucose absorbs water from your tissues, making you feel dehydrated and thirsty. Lots of water is also lost in the urine due to frequent urination, which again makes you dehydrated and thirsty.

Feeling more tired than usual

Sugar is body's main fuel. Though there is excess glucose in the blood, body cannot utilize it to produce energy and hence, you feel tired and weak.

Wounds and small injuries do not heal fast

High sugar level in the blood and tissues decreases body's ability to heal and fight infection. This leads to recurring infections and delayed wound healing. Even a small scratch can get infected and become big.

Overweight or loosing weight in spite of eating more

As told above since you feel more hungry, you may eat more than usual and gain weight. But the opposite also can occur. You may eat more than normal, but still lose weight because your body cannot use glucose to generate growth and energy. Weight loss happens more commonly in type 1 diabetes and weight gain in type 2 diabetes.

Burning, tingling and numbness in the feet

High blood sugar can damage nerves in the body. In the beginning small nerves in the feet get affected, hence, there may be burning, tingling, and numbness in the feet. Later on it may involve the legs and hands. If sugars are controlled these symptoms may disappear. If sugar remains uncontrolled for many years, nerve damage may become permanent.

Blurred vision

High levels of blood sugar can also get into the eye lens and change its refractory power, which can cause blurred vision. Once your diabetes is treated and your blood sugar levels become normal, vision should improve. However, if diabetes is uncontrolled for many years it can damage the retina, which is like a screen, and present in the back part of your eye. Severe damage to retina can lead to vision problems that are irreversible and may cause blindness.

Itching in the genital organs

This is also due to high blood sugars. Many fungal infections can develop in the genitals due to high sugar, which may cause itching.

Among the above complaints, increased thirst and frequent urination are more common. If a person has any of the above complaints, then his blood sugar should be tested. If you have a blood relative with diabetes, then it is even more reason to test your blood sugars. All these symptoms go off with treatment of diabetes. Since many of the above symptoms develop very slowly, they may go unnoticed for many months or years. Many people do not have any of the above symptoms even if they have diabetes and are picked up during a routine health check when their urine or blood sample is tested.

Do you have diabetes?

Go through the following questions to know whether you should get your blood sugar tested. If the answer is yes to any of the following questions, then get your blood sugar tested. Tell your family member or friend to get their blood sugar tested if their answer is also yes to any of the following questions. They will be very grateful to you for your help in detecting their diabetes early.

1. Do you have excessive thirst, excessive hunger, and pass large amount of urine?
2. Are you losing weight in spite of eating well?
3. Do you feel fatigued and tired all the time for no apparent reason?
4. Do you experience any tingling, numbness, or burning sensation in the hands and feet especially at night?
5. Do you get frequent infections?
6. Do you have any itching in genital area?
7. Does any injury, or wound, take a long time to heal?
8. Do you have any difficulty seeing or do you need to change glasses often?
9. Did you get cataracts at an early age?
10. Is your blood cholesterol high?
11. Do you have high blood pressure?
12. Do you have any heart problem especially at a young age?
13. Do you have any sexual problems such as impotency?
14. Are you overweight?
15. Does any of your blood relative has diabetes?
16. Do you have recurrent abortions or delivering large babies?
17. Are you pregnant?
18. Are you above 40 years of age?

Testing for blood sugar levels

Note that everyone has sugar in the blood. In fact, if the sugar level is too low we would not be able to live at all. What happens in a diabetic is that blood sugar is more than what is required. In a normal person, blood sugar levels are as follows.

Fasting blood glucose	— less than 110 mg/dl
Post prandial blood sugar	— less than 140 mg/dl
Random blood sugar	— less than 200 mg/dl

Earlier, urine glucose testing was being used to know whether a person has diabetes. But this is no longer recommended because many kidney diseases can lead to glucose leakage into urine even with normal blood sugars and urine may test positive for glucose. Hence, urine glucose testing alone should not be used to diagnose diabetes, but it can be used with blood tests.

An FBS (fasting blood sugar) measurement is the most convenient test after overnight fasting. It is called fasting sugar test, because you go for test on empty stomach. You should have your usual dinner and sleep. In the morning, give your blood for testing. You can have plain water in the morning but do not take anything else until you give your blood for test. After giving blood for test, you can have breakfast. You have diabetes if your FBS is 126 mg/dl or more. But confirm it once more the next day or any other day. If the next time also FBS is more than 126 mg/dl then definitely you have diabetes.

A PPBS (postprandial blood sugar) level more than 140 mg/dl also means that you have diabetes. You should give blood for PPBS 2 hours after breakfast or lunch or dinner. Testing after any meal is OK. Note that sometimes your fasting glucose level may be normal but your PPBS may be high which happens in early diabetes. Hence, if you check only FBS, diabetes may be missed. So whenever possible test both.

What about testing RBS (random blood sugar)? RBS means blood sugar tested at any time of the day without regard to meals. RBS gives only a rough indication about the presence of diabetes. A RBS level of more than 200 mg/dl indicates diabetes. But it should be confirmed by FBS and PPBS measurements.

Sometimes doctors may do a test known as OGTT (oral glucose tolerance test). OGTT is nothing but same as above tests but in more controlled conditions. It is not necessary to do it usually because testing FBS and PPBS can diagnose diabetes. It is more often done in pregnancy to diagnose pregnancy related diabetes, which is also known as gestational diabetes. OGTT is done after an overnight fast. In the morning instead of having your breakfast, you are given 75 gm glucose dissolved in water. Blood is tested for glucose levels after 1, 2, and 3 hours. If 2 hr blood glucose level is 200 mg/dl or more, it confirms diabetes.

There is one more test called glycoHb (HbA1c) which most of you are not aware. We know that we have red blood cells

(RBCs) in our blood, which live for about 3 months and die. There is something called hemoglobin (Hb) inside RBCs. Now the sugar in our blood and hemoglobin combine with each other to form a product called glycoHb. In normal persons, this glycoHb is less than 6.5. If blood sugar is high as in diabetes, more sugar will combine with hemoglobin and more glycoHb will be formed. GlycoHb gives an average of previous 3 months blood sugar since RBCs live for 3 months. This test is more expensive than FBS and PPBS, but very helpful to know how well sugars were controlled for the previous 3 months.

It was mentioned above that if a person has FBS value of 126 or more, then he has diabetes and if the FBS is less than 110 mg/dl then it is normal. Now, suppose a person has a FBS value between 100 and 126, then what about him? Is he normal or does he have diabetes? Answer is, he is having what is known as 'pre-diabetes' state. Another situation is FBS is normal but PPBS is 140–199 mg/dl. This is also called pre-diabetes state. People with these pre diabetic states have a relatively high risk of developing full-blown diabetes and should be treated with diet and exercise. They should get their blood sugar tested every year to know whether they have developed full diabetes.

3

Maintaining Normal Body Weight

Maintaining a normal body weight is an important aspect of maintaining good health. Being obese or overweight can lead to many problems. It is not just the question of looks. There are many diseases, which attack obese people more than lean people. Examples are high blood pressure (BP), diabetes, joint problems, heart diseases etc.

How to know whether you have normal body weight

You should know whether you are normal body weight or overweight or obese. People are of different heights and different heights have different weights. Both weight and height are important to know whether a person has normal bodyweight.

METHOD-1. KNOWING YOUR IDEAL BODY WEIGHT USING BMI.

There is something called "body mass index" (BMI) which takes into account both height and weight. A person with normal body weight has a BMI of 18.5-24.9. By knowing your BMI, you can know whether you have normal body weight or not.

BMI Categories:

- Underweight = <18.5
- Normal weight = 18.5-24.9
- Overweight = 25-29.9
- Obesity = BMI of 30 or greater

How to calculate your BMI (Body Mass Index)

There is a very simple formula to calculate your BMI. You require two things to know your BMI. These two things are your weight in kgs and height in meters. The formula to calculate BMI is

$$BMI = \frac{\text{Weight (in kgs)}}{\text{Height}^2 \text{ (in meters)}}$$

Example: suppose your weight is 60 kgs and height is 160 cms (i.e. 1.6 meters). Your BMI would be,

$$BMI = 60/ (1.6)^2$$

$$\text{i.e.} \quad = 60/ 2.56 = 23.4$$

Therefore, your BMI would be 23.4, which is normal.

METHOD-2. KNOWING YOUR IDEAL BODY WEIGHT USING YOUR HEIGHT.

This is a simple way to find out one's ideal body weight. For this, it is enough to know your height in cms.

The formula is,

Ideal body weight = Height (in cms.) - 100

Suppose your height is 160 cms,

Your ideal body weight should be 160 – 100 = 60 kgs.

METHOD-3. KNOWING YOUR IDEAL BODY WEIGHT USING YOUR HEIGHT.

Another way to know what your ideal weight should be is to measure your height in cms and look at the following charts.

Ideal Weight Chart for Men

Height (centimeters)	*Small frame (weight in kgs)*	*Medium frame (weight in kgs)*	*Large frame (weight in kgs)*
157.5	58.1-60.8	59.4-64.0	62.6-68.0
160.0	59.0-61.7	60.3-64.9	63.5-69.4
162.6	59.9-62.6	61.2-65.8	64.4-70.7
165.1	60.8-63.5	62.1-67.1	65.3-72.6
167.6	61.7-64.4	63.0-68.5	66.2-74.4
170.2	62.6-65.8	64.4-69.8	67.6-76.2
172.7	63.5-67.1	65.8-71.2	68.9-78.0
175.3	64.4-68.5	67.1-72.6	70.3-79.8
177.8	65.3-69.8	68.5-73.9	71.7-81.6
180.3	66.2-71.2	69.8-75.3	73.0-83.5

182.9	67.6-72.6	71.2-77.1	74.4-85.3
185.4	68.9-74.4	72.6-78.9	76.2-87.1
188.0	70.3-76.2	74.4-80.7	78.0-89.4
190.5	71.7-78.0	75.7-82.6	79.8-91.6
193.0	73.5-79.8	77.6-84.8	82.1-93.9

Ideal Weight Chart for Women

Height (centimeters)	*Small frame (weight in kgs)*	*Medium frame (weight in kgs)*	*Large frame (weight in kgs)*
147.3	45.9-49.9	49.0-54.0	53.1-58.9
149.9	46.3-50.8	49.9-55.3	54.0-60.3
152.4	46.8-51.7	50.8-56.7	54.9-61.6
154.9	47.7-53.1	51.7-58.0	56.2-63.0
157.5	48.6-54.4	53.1-59.4	57.6-64.3
160.0	49.9-55.8	54.4-60.7	58.9-66.1
162.6	51.3-57.1	55.8-62.1	66.3-67.9
165.1	52.6-58.5	57.1-63.4	61.6-69.7
167.6	54.0-59.8	58.5-64.8	63.0-71.5
170.2	55.3-61.2	59.3-66.1	64.3-73.3
172.7	56.7-62.5	61.2-67.5	65.7-75.4
175.3	58.5-63.9	62.5-68.8	67.5-76.5
177.8	59.4-65.2	63.9-70.2	68.4-77.8
180.3	60.7-66.6	65.2-71.5	69.7-79.2
182.9	62.1-67.9	66.6-72.9	71.1-80.5

By using any of the above methods, you can know whether you have normal weight or not. If you are overweight or obese, you need to reduce your weight. To reduce your weight, try to control your food, do exercise, improve your lifestyle. Excess body weight means more fat in the body. More fat in the body means more diseases and complications as told earlier. Achieving ideal body weight (or BMI) can prevent all these, and can reduce the severity of diseases like high BP and diabetes. In fact many people

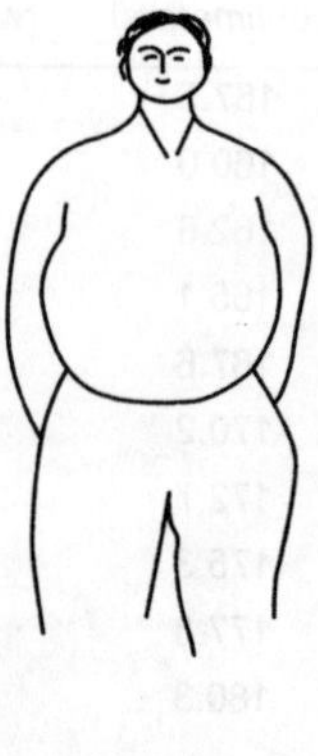

are able to cure their diabetes (early stages) simply by achieving normal body weight.

What to do if your body weight is not ideal

You should try to achieve the ideal weight for your height. Achieving ideal weight depends on the way you eat. Or to say it in scientific terms, your weight depends on the amount of calories you eat. Calories are nothing but the amount of energy available in foods. Your weight depends on the balance between the amount of calories that you take and the amount of calories you spend. All of us do some activity daily and we need to spend calories for these activities. If the amount of calories that you take is more than the amount you spend, you will put on weight. If the amount of calories that you spend is more than the amount you eat, then you will lose weight. This is like a bank balance. If you spend, more than you credit into your account there will be negative bank balance. If you spend less and credit more, there will be positive bank balance. The total number of calories that you need to eat per day will depend on what your present weight is and what your ideal weight should be.

Look at the following chart to know how much food you should take depending on your weight.

Normal Weight	*Underweight*	*Overweight*
Continue your usual amount of food	You can increase your food intake	You need to reduce your food intake

Roughly, if you eat 7700 calories more than you spend; you will put on one Kilogram of body weight. On the other hand, if you spend 7700 calories more than you eat by doing exercise or any other physical work, you will lose one kilogram of weight.

Now, can you eat 7700 calories in one day to put on 1 kg weight or can you spend 7700 calories in one day (by doing heavy exercise) to lose 1 kg weight. The answer is NO, because 7700 calories is a huge amount to eat or spend in one or two days. In fact, a normal person's total daily food intake is a total of 1500-2500 calories per day. Here, you have to remember one important thing. Do not be overenthusiastic and struggle to lose weight within a short period. You should lose weight gradually and losing about 1.5 to 2 kilograms every month is a good target. This works out to a reduction of 250 to 300 calories per day.

If you try to lose weight rapidly, you will have to drastically cut down your diet, and exercise rigorously. Though in the beginning you may follow it for a while, it is difficult to maintain such a rigid diet and exercise regimen for a long period. The result is that you might lose weight rapidly initially, but you will soon go back to your old schedule and regain the lost weight. Then after a while, it is back to the rigid diet and exercise schedule. This happens often to many people and is called the Yo-Yo phenomenon, where the weight goes up and down in cycles.

If you have a normal body weight, then continue with your usual amount of food. All that you have to do is cut down on sugar and unhealthy foods. Many diabetics have less than normal body weight. Though having less body weight is not as dangerous as more body weight, still it is advantageous to have normal body weight. Underweight diabetics may not be able to put up enough resistance against infections. If you are underweight, slightly increase your food intake to gain some weight. Here again, increase your calories slowly and aim for a slow and gradual weight gain. But note that all the principles of diabetic diet still apply to you and you should not increase sugar and fat intake.

4 Changing your Lifestyle

Lifestyle means the way you live your life. It includes the way you eat, the way you work and exercise, the way you sleep, the way you think and your habits. There is good lifestyle and there is bad lifestyle. Good lifestyle makes you healthy and bad lifestyle brings you diseases. Most of the diseases, including diabetes can be prevented if you cultivate a good lifestyle. Healthy lifestyle is very important in managing diseases like high BP, diabetes and heart problems. There are many people who could have easily lived around 100 years but die early at their forties and fifties because of their bad lifestyle.

Good Lifestyle

Good lifestyle is the one, which makes you healthy. A good lifestyle consists of the following.

Right eating

Eat more of healthy foods like vegetables and foods of plant origin. Cut down non-veg, oils and fats. Eat in moderation. Avoid overeating and under eating. It is said that digestive power is like fire. Just as fire is put off by both too much of firewood and too little firewood, digestive fire is also put off by too much or too little food. Eat only when you are hungry, because when you are hungry your digestive system is very active. If you eat when not hungry, food is not digested properly and the body cannot get proper nourishment. Many people go by clock and eat even if they are not hungry which is wrong.

Right activity

Avoid sedentary lifestyle i.e. sitting in one place and not doing much bodily work. Your job may require you to sit in one place like office job, bank jobs etc. but after your office work, try to engage yourself in some physical activity. Activity can be anything. You need not go to gym and start lifting weights. Doing household activities like washing, cleaning and simple walking can bring you so many benefits. There are so many activities to choose from like walking, jogging, tennis, yoga, swimming, and aerobic exercises.

Right habits

Right habits bring out your creative potential and contribute to your personal growth. Good habits include painting, music, reading, or learning some new skill. Bad habits destroy your mental and physical health and include smoking, drinking alcohol, chewing tobacco etc. If you are smoking and drinking alcohol first stop it. It is like committing a slow suicide. If you are smoking, you are more likely to develop a cancer, high BP, heart attacks, and strokes. If you are drinking alcohol, you are more likely to develop liver damage, brain damage, and depression. People smoke, drink and they think they are relaxing or solving a problem. This is wrong. All that happens is more problems build up and existing problems get postponed. Problems are never solved by smoking and drinking.

Dangers of smoking

- Bad breath, gum disease and stained teeth
- Decreased energy and tiredness
- You get irritated and angry fast
- High blood pressure
- Unnecessary expenditure
- Risk of lung cancer and many other types of cancer
- High risk of heart attack and stroke
- Lung problems like cough and breathing problems
- More wrinkles. You look more aged
- Risk of stomach ulcers and acidity
- Risk of damage to babies if pregnant women smoke

If you cannot quit smoking and drinking yourself take help from your doctor. There are many methods and medicines to help you quit smoking and drinking. If you are not successful once, do not get disappointed. Keep trying. Keep a diary with you and write down the situations and reasons, which bring the urge in you to smoke. This diary can help both you and your doctor understand your smoking better and plan methods to quit. Never keep cigarettes in your pocket and at home. Availability makes you smoke more. Whenever you feel the urge to smoke, divert your attention to something else, like reading a magazine or newspaper, going for a walk, watching TV, playing with children, sipping a cup of tea or coffee or eating a chocolate.

Cigarettes mainly contain nicotine and it is because of nicotine you feel the kick and urge. There are many preparations of nicotine available in medical stores in the form of chewing gum, patch, nasal spray, inhaler and lozenges. You can buy one of these from a medical store. But first talk to your doctor whether you should use them. Whenever you feel the urge to smoke, instead of smoking, you can chew a nicotine gum. This will bring down your urge without making you smoke. However, you cannot go on using nicotine replacements indefinitely. That also needs to be stopped once you feel more confident as a nonsmoker. It is like removing a thorn with another thorn but ultimately both have to be thrown.

Right thinking

Do not have negative thoughts. Always think positively. Negative emotions like jealousy, hatred, greed, excessive anger are all bad for your physical and mental health. Positive emotions like love, sympathy etc. have been proven to have positive effect on your health. Do some meditation and relaxation, read some spiritual books. Keep your morale high.

So why wait? Change your lifestyle today

A good lifestyle will bestow you both physical and mental health. Many diseases will not even touch you. If you already have some disease like diabetes, it may just disappear or will come under good control. A good lifestyle is necessary for everyone. So look into your lifestyle today. If it is good, then congratulations. If it is bad, change it today!

5 Managing Diabetes with Diet

We are what we eat. Food has such a direct effect on our body and mind, that all of us need to pay great attention to what we eat, how much we eat and how we eat.

A good diet not only controls your blood sugar but also controls your weight, blood pressure, cholesterol and also improves your health. A good diet also reduces the chances of developing stroke, heart attacks and joint problems. Being a diabetic you need to know what is good and what is bad for you, what to eat what to avoid. Learning to eat healthy food is an important part of your diabetes management.

Many people think that a diabetic has to give up many of his favorite foods. Having to take sugarless drinks like coffee, tea and unable to eat sweets is a nightmare for many. Though this is true to some extent, still you can enjoy most of your food even if you are a diabetic. There is no need to eat only bland, boring foods. You can eat a variety of foods. Only thing is, you need to eat more vegetables, whole grains, foods that are high in nutrition and low in calories, fewer animal products and fats.

All our food items can be groped mainly into 7 groups;

	Food Group	*Examples*
1	Cereals	Rice, wheat, jowar
2	Vegetables	Cabbage, tomato
3	Milk	Cow milk, curds
4	Meats	Chicken, fish
5	Fruits	Apple, banana
6	Fats/Oils	Ghee, butter, cheese
7	Pulses/Dals	Bengal gram, dal

Our daily food consists of items from some or all the above groups. Every food item is made of mainly 3 components; carbohydrates, proteins and fats. But the proportion of these 3 components is different in different food items. For example, meat is rich in protein, rice is rich in carbohydrates, and ghee is rich in fat. Now let us learn something about these three components.

Carbohydrates. Carbohydrates turn into glucose very fast in the body. They provide energy required by the body. Carbohydrates are found in fruits, vegetables, rice, ragi, wheat, jowar, dairy foods, and breads.

Protein. Protein is found in eggs, meat, poultry, fish, dairy products, and beans. Proteins are the building blocks of our body especially muscles.

Fat. Butter, ghee, margarine, and oils are fats. Fat is also found in many dairy and meat products like pork. Fat is also a good source of energy but usually we use carbohydrates for our energy requirement. Excess fat gets deposited under the skin and causes obesity. Cholesterol, which is a type of fat, can get deposited inside blood vessels and block them leading to many problems.

Usually carbohydrates make up 70% of our food. Carbohydrates have highest impact on blood sugar level because they get absorbed from the intestine fast. If you eat more carbohydrates, blood sugar level can go high. Hence, you need to keep track of carbohydrates that you eat. You need not eat less quantity of food to do this. All that you have to do is to eat more proteins and vegetables instead of carbohydrates. Instead of eating large amounts of carbohydrates at one time eat less quantity each time but more times. Proteins have less impact on blood sugar. They do not raise the blood sugar fast. Fat also does not cause fast rise in blood sugar but excess fat is not good for health.

Eat healthy foods

Healthy foods are those, which are close to nature, have lots of vitamins, minerals, roughage and contain less of fat and cholesterol. Processed, canned, or frozen foods that contain artificial additives and lots of fat can be called unhealthy foods. Some tips about choosing healthy foods are as follows:

- Include lots of vegetables in your food.
- Fruits are rich in vitamins and minerals. Taking small amount of fruits (one fruit per day) does not increase your blood sugar and is good for your health.
- Keep oils and fats to minimum. They contain lots of unsaturated fats and cholesterol, which are not good for you. They may get collected in blood vessels and block them, causing heart attacks, strokes, and gangrene.
- Use salt in moderate amounts. Do not add extra salt to your food. Also, avoid canned and boxed foods as they may contain lots of salt.
- Cut down non-veg food. Man is a born vegetarian. Eating non-veg is a learned habit. Research shows that our teeth and digestive system are made to eat and digest veg food, not non-veg food. But then, don't be guilty of eating non-veg what I am saying is cut down, don't make non-veg your main diet.

Do not think that eating healthy foods means you should not eat other foods. Other foods can also be eaten, but less frequently. There are what are known as food pyramids, which can help you decide what to eat more and what to eat less. One such pyramid developed by U.S. Department of Agriculture and supported by the Department of Health and Human Services is shown here. It outlines what to eat more and what to eat less, but it is not a rigid prescription. Foods, which you should eat more, are in the base of the pyramid. As you go up towards the tip, there are foods which you should eat less frequently. You can use it as a general guide in choosing a healthy diet that is right for you. A food guide pyramid is shown in Fig. 5.1.

Eat your meals regularly

Being a diabetic you need to eat your meals regularly if you are taking treatment, which may be tablets, insulin or both. Suppose you take your tablets or insulin in the morning and skip lunch you may develop low blood sugar, which can be dangerous. Try to eat at the same time everyday. Eating lunch at 1 pm on one

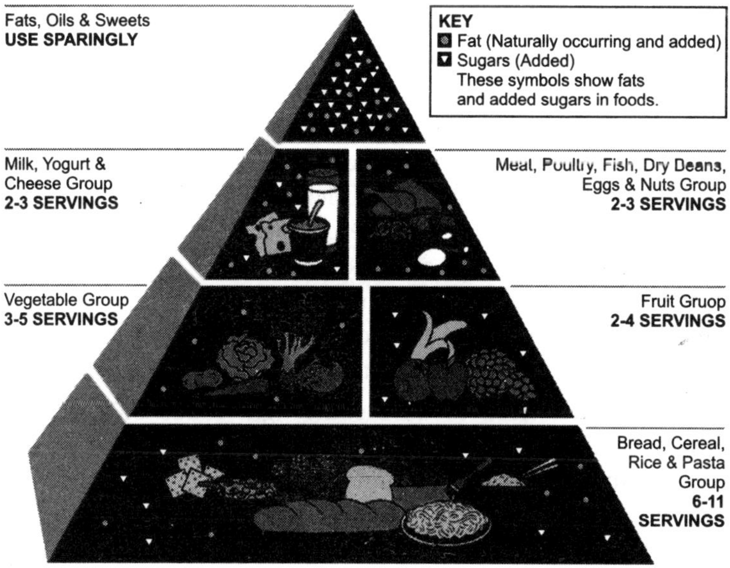

Source: U.S. Department of Agriculture

Fig. 5.1: Food pyramid

day and at 3 pm, another day is to be avoided. Small changes are OK, but proponing or postponing by many hours is to be avoided. You also need to be consistent with your diet i.e. try to eat the same quantity of food everyday. Eating more on one day and less another day is not good because this may cause erratic blood sugar levels. Blood sugar becomes high when you eat more and low when you eat less. If you eat a big lunch at one time and small lunch at another time, then your blood sugar level becomes erratic. When you eat more, it becomes more and when you eat less, blood sugar becomes less. If you eat a light breakfast everyday, keep it same everyday. If you eat big lunch, keep it same everyday. Same does not mean that it should be exactly same, it should be roughly same. You may also develop hypoglycemia (low blood sugar level) if you take the same amount of tablets or insulin but eat less. Delayed or missed meals are one of the most common causes of hypoglycemia. If you think you are not going to have your usual meal, then it is better to skip the dose of insulin or tablet which you take before that meal.

If you are taking tablets to control your diabetes, then try to eat the same quantity of food daily at regular times. Also, take the tablets at the times prescribed. Taking a tablet before, with, or after meals can have different effects on your blood sugar level. Consistency with the quantity and timing is all the more important if you are taking insulin. You cannot eat whenever you want after taking insulin. For example, after taking human insulin you should wait 20 – 30 minutes and then have food unless your doctor told you otherwise.

All diabetics need to have some light foods or snacks in between major meals to prevent hypoglycemia, which usually develops in between the meals if you are on empty stomach. A bedtime snack is also very important for all diabetics who take insulin injections. This ensures that blood glucose level does not become low during the night especially midnight.

You should also have some snacks before exercising and before any unexpected physical activity. For example, you may have to walk unexpectedly due to some reason. That time it is better to have some light snacks and proceed. This will prevent exercise-induced hypoglycemia.

What food can you eat?

You can eat the same food that you used to eat before you had diabetes with some changes. You can eat a breakfast, eat a snack at around 10-30 to 11 am, a lunch, an evening snack and a dinner. All that you have to remember is to cut down on sweets, oily and fried foods. Also, avoid excess salt because excess salt can increase your BP. Include more vegetables. It is not necessary to buy special diabetic foods, which are expensive and give no additional benefit to you other than your regular food.

A diet sheet (you can obtain one from your doctor or dietician) can help you in choosing the right food in right quantity. Sometimes it is difficult to keep track of how much carbohydrates, proteins, and calories you are eating. A general rule is that if you are overweight, eat whatever you were eating before, but less quantity (of course with the changes mentioned earlier). If you are not sure what to eat and how much to eat, take the help of a registered dietitian to help you put together a meal plan that fits your health goals, food preferences and lifestyle. The most important thing to follow is consistency with your meal plan. Once you have decided on a meal plan, try to eat the same amount of food with the same proportion of carbohydrates, proteins, and fats at the same time every day. This will keep your blood sugar at a consistent level.

Carbohydrates should make 70% of you diet. Foods with high carbohydrate content include bread, cereals (rice, ragi, wheat, jowar etc), beans, fruits, and vegetables. Fruits and vegetables contain lots of fiber, which is good to prevent constipation and cut down calories. High fiber diet is recommended for all and not only for diabetics. Take less of high calorie and low nutritional value foods, such as chocolates.

Keep protein intake in the range of 15-20% of total calories. Choose protein foods, which are low in fat such as nonfat dairy products, legumes, skinless poultry, eggs, fish and lean meats. Example of a protein food with high fat is pork. The yellow part of egg contains more cholesterol so it is good idea to eat only the white part and discard yellow part, especially if your cholesterol level is high.

Reduce the amount of dietary fat to 10-15% of total calories. The current American Diabetes association guidelines advise that less than 7-10% of calories should come from saturated fat. These are the fats that raise LDL ("bad") cholesterol. Unsaturated fat is better than saturated fat. Example of unsaturated fat is sunflower oil. Example of saturated fat is dalda, butter, animal fat like pork fat. Eating fewer fats not only decreases your cholesterol levels but also helps in decreasing your body weight.

Sometimes sticking on to your meal plan is difficult. It is OK if you cannot follow dietary rules occasionally. But try to stay motivated and eat in the healthiest way possible.

Avoid the following foods or keep them to minimum

- Alcohol
- Cakes
- Chocolate
- Fruit juice concentrate
- Glucose
- Glucose drinks
- Honey
- Ice cream
- Jam
- Lactose
- Maltose
- Molasses
- Pudding
- Sugar
- Sweet biscuits
- Sweets of all kinds

Eat in moderate quantity

- Bread rolls
- Breads
- Chicken
- Dried fruits
- Foods containing flour like idly, dosa
- Fruit juice without sugar
- Milk foods
- Mutton
- Potatoes
- Thick soups
- Wheat flour
- Yam

Can eat little freely

- Cabbage
- Cauliflower
- Clear soups
- Fresh lime juice without sugar
- Greens
- Pepper
- Salads
- Small onions
- Spices
- Tea or coffee without sugar with skimmed milk
- Thin fishes

List of vegetables that may be taken

- Ashgourd
- Banana flower
- Banana stem
- Bitter gourd
- Brinjals
- Cabbage
- Cauli flower
- Drumstick
- Karamani beans
- Ladies finger
- Noil koil
- Snake gourd
- Tender beans
- Tomatoes

List of fruits that may be taken (one friut per day)

Fruit	Quantity	Fruit	Quantity
• Apple	1 small	• Mango	1 small
• Apricots	2 fresh	• Melon	1 slice
• Banana	½ small	• Orange	1 average
• Custard apple	1 small	• Papaya	2-2 inchs slice
• Dates	2 no	• Peach	1 medium
• Grape fruits	20 no	• Pear	1 small
• Guava	1 medium size	• Pineapple	1 slice
• Indian gooseberry	1-2 no	• Plums	2
		• Sapota	1 small
• Jack fruit	3 piece	• Sweet lime	1 medium size
• Jambu	10 small	• Yellow grapes	10 no

Use more of

- Bengal gram
- Bitter gourd
- Black gram
- Carry leaves
- Coriander leaves
- Fenugreek leaves
- Fenugreek seeds
- Lettuce
- Soya bean
- Spinach
- Tomato

(Courtesy, food list: Diet department, Kasturba Hospital, Manipal)

Can you take sugar?

Almost all diabetics think that they should not take sugar. Diabetics are routinely advised not to add sugar to tea, coffee, etc. In fact, it is a universal practice not to add sugar to coffee, tea etc. Though not adding sugar to drinks is a good way of cutting down calories, here is happy and surprising news for you. You can actually add sugar to your tea, coffee etc. In recent years, it has been shown that eating some sugar does not usually cause problems for most people with diabetes—as long as it does not increase the total amount of calories consumed and is part of a balanced diet. If you take sugar, subtract the amount of carbohydrates form somewhere else. For example if you add 15 gms sugar to your tea, do not eat half chapatti that day. This will keep the total amount of calories same. Of course eating too much sugar will increase your blood sugar. However, adding small amount of sugar to your tea or coffee does not affect your blood sugar. Do not think sugar as your enemy. You should carry some sugar, sweet or chocolate in your pocket always. Eating them when you develop low blood sugar will normalize sugar level. Eating sugar or sweets is necessary when you develop low blood sugar levels.

Can you take alcohol?

There is no simple answer for this. Today drinking has become an accepted social custom. Though it is better for the diabetic to avoid alcohol, let us be more practical and say if you have to drink, then drink sparingly and sensibly.

Though most alcoholic drinks do not have vitamins, proteins, or fats, they do contain good amount of calories, which will have to be counted in the total number of calories that is permitted per day. 1 gram of alcohol gives seven calories. You can easily calculate the total number of calories in the drink by the following formula.

0.4 × proof × number of ounces = calories

The "proof" is double the alcohol percentage, i.e. 12% alcohol content means 24 proof. Percentage of alcohol content is mentioned on the bottles.

A bottle of beer (650 ml) gives about 400-500 calories, which is a huge amount. Wines, in addition to alcohol, also contain sugars, which add to the calories. Drinks like whisky, rum vodka, gin, etc, contain around 80 calories per ounce (30 ml). People usually have snacks along with alcohol, which can also add up to too many calories. It is important for a diabetic to avoid fried and oily snacks and instead eat a salad of raw vegetables like carrots, cucumbers etc along with drinks. You need to cut down other foods to compensate for the excess calories provided by alcohol.

There are some dangers involved when a diabetic takes alcohol. Hypoglycemia (low blood sugar) can happen after taking excessive alcohol because alcohol can stop the liver from making glucose. Drinking can also mask the signs and symptoms of hypoglycemia so that the person has no warning of the attack and may suddenly become unconscious. Therefore, it is important to take only a limited amount of alcohol and food should not be skipped after the alcohol intake. Diabetics who are on sulfonylureas, especially chlorpropamide (not used now a days), may experience an acute reaction when they drink alcohol. There is usually flushing of face, choking sensation, nausea, vomiting and headache. Sometimes blood pressure may become low. Diabetics who are taking biguanides like phenformin and metformin may develop an other problem called lactic acidosis, which is a serious condition (see chapter 17) with the use of alcohol. 1 in 2 persons with lactic acidosis die even with best treatment. Hence, a diabetic who is on phenformin or metformin should avoid taking alcohol. Therefore, if the diabetic feels it a necessity to drink, he should take alcohol sparingly and sensibly! May be not more than 1 or 2 pegs at a time.

Artificial sweeteners

Artificial sweeteners are low in calories and include aspartame, neotame, saccharin, and sucralose. These artificial sweeteners are safe and can be taken by all people, including people with diabetes and pregnant women. Artificial sweeteners contain half the calories as compare to natural sugar and cause lesser rise in blood sugar after eating. They not only help you in weight and sugar control but can also add taste to your tea, coffee etc. If you are bored of sipping sugarless tea, coffee etc, you can buy one of these products.

Glycaemic index

Different types of foods are digested at different rates and therefore have different effects in terms of raising blood sugar level after a meal. Some foods are rapidly digested to glucose (e.g. cornflakes), while others are digested slowly and it takes more time for the glucose to reach the bloodstream (e.g. rotis). Glycemic index quantifies the effect of different foods on blood sugar level. Higher the glycemic index, higher is the rise in blood sugar after eating that food. So a diabetic person should eat more of low glycemic index foods and avoid high glycemic index foods.

Dietary supplements

A dietary supplement is a product taken by mouth that contains a "dietary ingredient" intended to supplement the diet. These dietary supplements may include vitamins, minerals, herbs or other botanicals, proteins, and substances such as enzymes etc. Dietary supplements may come in the form of tablets, capsules, powders, liquids etc. Many supplements contain active ingredients that have strong biological effects and their safety is not always assured in all users. Some supplements may interact with your daily medicines. You need to be careful before you buy any dietary supplement on your own. Most of the time you do not need any dietary supplement like multivitamin tablets if you are having nutritious food daily. So do not take supplements on your own. Consult your doctor before taking them. If you need any supplements, he should decide about it.

Food exchanges

Food exchanges are nothing but eating one type of food instead of other type. If you are getting bored with one type of food, you may want to eat some other type of food without increasing the number of calories you eat. By looking at the food exchange list, you can choose some other food with the same amount of calories. For example if you are bored of eating bread, instead of eating bread you can exchange with a vegetable. One slice of bread is equal to half-cup vegetables in terms of calories. So you can eat half cup vegetables instead of one slice bread and keep the number of calories same. A sample food exchange list is given below. You can choose a variety of foods by looking at the charts given in appendix-I.

Sample Exchange List

Food group	*You can have.....*	*Or exchange it for...*
Cereals	1 large slice or 2 small slice (provides 80 calories)	1 chapatti (6 inches size) or ½ cup vegetables 1 dosa (10 inches size)
Fruit	1 apple, two inch wide (provides 60 calories)	½ banana (9 inches long) or 1 cup cooked vegetables
Vegetable	1 cup cooked vegetables (provides 56 calories)	2 cup mixed salad or 3/4th of a chapatti or 1½-cup vegetable juice.

Sugar	1 teaspoon	1/3rd chapatti
Milk	1 cup milk	1 cup cooked dal or chana or 1½-cup cooked vegetables
Meat	30 gms of meat, fish, poultry	1/2 cup dried beans
Fat	1 teaspoon oil, butter or margarine	½ cup milk or ½ chapatti

Making use of food labels to improve your diet planning

Now-a-days most of the readymade packed and bottled foods carry what is known as food label. Food label is nothing but the information printed on the food about the amount of carbohydrates, proteins, fats, and calories. The amount of carbohydrate, which is usually given in grams, helps in carbohydrate counting. The listing of protein in gms can give you an idea about how much protein you are having. It is helpful to know the protein content especially for people with kidney damage. People with kidney damage need to cut down on protein intake because protein gets converted to urea in the body which cannot be removed by damaged kidneys.

How much to eat

There are many things to consider while deciding how much to eat. Your weight, your work, etc should be considered to decide how much you should eat.

If you are normal weight for your height, you can continue with your usual amount of food. If you are a heavy worker, you need to eat more food than a person who works less. An office worker who sits most of the time requires fewer calories than a farmer who works in fields. For children with diabetes (usually type 1 diabetes), it is important to give adequate food to support their natural growth and development. The usual rules of dieting do not apply to them, though a healthy and nutritious diet is also important to them. Do not withhold food when the child is hungry and do not force the child to eat if not hungry. On special occasions (like birthdays or festivals), you need to plan more because you may eat more food on such occasions including sweets. You need not deny yourself the pleasure of eating sweets on such occasions. All that you have to do is see that you eat fewer carbohydrates on that day. For example, if birthday cake, ice cream or other sweets are eaten, then decrease the amount of other carbohydrate foods such as potatoes, chapattis, or rice. Such substitution allows you to eat what you want and keeps the total number of calories more or less the same.

If you are a type 2 diabetic, you are most likely to be overweight, and need to eat a diet that helps you lose weight. 80% to 90% of people with type 2 diabetes are overweight. How much weight to lose depends on how much overweight you are. In many cases, moderate weight loss and increased physical activity can control type 2 diabetes even without medicines.

Some sample recommendations for how much you should eat

Your profile	*How many calories you should have*
A small woman who exercises	1200 – 1600
A small or medium woman who wants to lose weight	1200 – 1600
A medium woman who does not exercise much	1200 – 1600
A large woman who wants to lose weight	1600 – 2000
A large woman who exercises a lot or has a physically active job	2000 – 2400
A small man with normal weight	1600 – 2000
A medium man who does not exercise much	1600 – 2000
A medium to large man who wants to lose weight	1600 – 2000
A medium/large man who does a lot of exercise or has a physically active job	2000 – 2400
A large man with normal weight	2000 – 2400

Measuring food items

You must have seen a diabetic diet chart. There are so many measurements like ounce, gms, cups etc. The problem for everyone is how to measure food items. Most people are uncomfortable measuring food items. Even simple measures like cups and spoons can mean so many things, because there are cups and spoons of so many sizes. To be frank, it is not practical to weigh each food and then start eating it. But if you want to be accurate, there is no way other than weighing each food item and then calculating its calorie content. Within a few days, you will get a very good visual grasp of the amounts and will not really have to bother about the precise weights and volumes. Try to remember the following measurements.

1 ounce = 30 gms = 30 ml
1 teaspoon = 5 ml
1 tablespoon = 15 ml
1 cup = 240 ml = 8 fl. Ounces

Summarizing the diabetic diet advice —Points to Remember

- Eat a variety of foods every day, such as starches, vegetables, fruits, milk and yogurt.
- Limit the amounts of fats and sweets you eat each day.
- Choose the amount of food carefully depending on your body weight. Take the help of your doctor or dietician for this.
- Eat about the same amount of food each day.
- Eat at about the same time each day.
- Cut down alcohol intake or better still stop drinking.

6 Managing Diabetes with Exercise

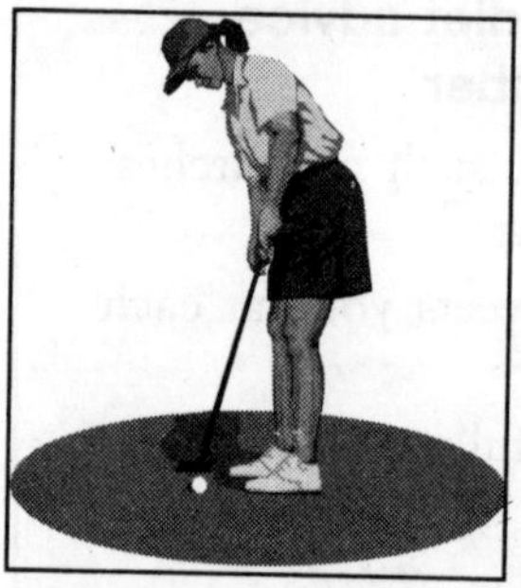

To rest is to rust. Our body is designed to work and be active. An inactive person becomes a home to many diseases just as stagnant water becomes home to many worms and bacteria. Regular exercise is important not only for diabetics but also for everyone. Regular exercise helps in controlling blood sugar, helps burn excess calories and fat to achieve optimal weight. Exercise keeps you mentally healthy also. Exercise improves overall health. It decreases insulin resistance even without weight loss. Exercise also increases the body's energy level, lowers tension, and improves your ability to handle stress. Ancient physicians knew the fact that exercise helps in the treatment of diabetes. Both Charaka and Sushruta, two great ancient Indian physicians advocated the use of exercise in treating diabetes more than 2000 years ago. Following are the benefits of exercise:

- You feel more energetic
- Your digestion will improve
- Decreases backache and other joint pains
- Less stress
- Better self-esteem and mood
- Better sleep
- Good figure
- Controls your blood pressure
- Lowers blood glucose

- Lowers cholesterol level
- Heart and lungs become more healthy
- You live longer

What exercises should you do?

You need not join an expensive gymnasium and start working there. Take into consideration your job schedule and plan an exercise program. All that you need is simple exercise program like walking, jogging, cycling, biking, tennis, badminton, and swimming. Most of the exercises can be done at home. Yoga and pranayama are also very good for your physical and mental health.

Anybody can start doing exercises unless there is some major health problem like heart failure. If you have any such serious disease, consult your doctor to know what type and how much exercise is good for you. Activities like walking, jogging, and cycling can be done by most people. Always start slowly and build up your exercise program gradually. Aerobic exercises are good for everyone and are better than weight lifting exercises.

If you are walking daily, note down a certain distance from your house. Choose an area which is calm and without much traffic. First note down how much time it takes to cover the distance if you walk at your normal speed. Then gradually increase the speed of walking so that you can cover the same distance in a shorter time. Increase the speed of walking until you reach the maximum tolerated limit. After this, you can increase the distance of walking slowly. In the beginning, walking for about 15 minutes is O.K. increase this after a week to 20 minutes. Increase by 5 to 10 minutes every week so that by the end of 3 months you should be able to walk for 1 hour. If you are doing other exercises also, then you can cut down your walking duration accordingly.

Some important considerations before you start exercising

Though exercise is good for everyone, there are some basic things which you should be aware of especially if you are a diabetic.

The aim of your exercise is to train your body and not strain it! Always build up your exercise program slowly until you reach your targeted level of intensity. There are many overenthusiastic people who join a gym and start lifting heavy weights straightaway. This is dangerous, as your body may not tolerate sudden, vigorous exercise. Do not exercise beyond your capacity. Exercising too much can cause injuries to joints, muscles, and feet. Developing aches and pains in the body indicates that you have suddenly started with high intensity exercises.

Exercise involving heavy weights may be bad for people with high blood pressure, blood vessel disease, or eye problems. If you have diabetic proliferative retinopathy, you need to avoid strenuous exercises and certain yoga postures like shirshasana. Proliferative retinopathy is a condition where lots of weak blood vessels grow in the retina. These weak blood vessels may rupture and cause bleeding inside the eye when there is sudden rise in pressure inside them either due to strenuous exercises or due to headstand yoga postures. Any patient who has a severe degree of proliferative retinopathy should get the eyes treated with laser therapy before starting any exercise. You can know whether you have retinopathy during eye check up. However, you can start and continue mild forms of exercises like walking and aerobics.

Exercise can change the requirement for your medicines. you may require less tablets or insulin. If you are not accustomed to physical activity, start first with small exercises like walking and then gradually build up. As you become stronger, you can exercise more and more. Do some physical activity every day. It is better to walk 10 or 20 minutes each day than one hour once a week.

There is no problem if you are doing mild to moderate physical activities like walking, jogging, cycling, and other simple aerobic exercises. But if you want to do more exercise then you need to be careful and get advice from your doctor about how much exercise is good for you. If you have any heart problem, problems with your joints, backbone, feet etc then get your doctor's advice before doing exercise. If you have diabetes-related nerve damage, you need to be more careful because small injuries can go unnoticed and lead to more serious problems.

Exercise can lower your blood glucose. That is good and that is why you should do exercise. But it can become very low sometimes especially if you are taking insulin or oral medicines. Hypoglycemia can happen at the time you are exercising, just afterward, or even up to a day later. To prevent hypoglycemia during physical activity, it is good idea to check your blood sugar before and during any heavy exercise and if you experience any symptoms of hypoglycemia. You should not do exercise when your blood sugar is low or very high i.e. less than 80 or more than 300. If your blood sugar is low, eat a snack and then start your exercise. Do not skip any meals before exercise. It is always wise to carry some sugar, sweets, or chocolates with you when you exercise. After you finish exercise, check your blood sugar to see how it has affected your blood glucose level. If the exercise causes your blood sugar to drop very low, then you need to get your insulin or tablets adjusted by your doctor. Drink plenty of fluids during physical activity, to prevent dehydration.

Wear good cotton socks and well fitting soft shoes while exercising to prevent any possible injury to your feet. Wear loose, porous and preferably cotton clothes during exercise. Never walk or jog barefoot. After you exercise, it is good idea to check your feet for sores, blisters, irritation, cuts, or other injuries. If there are any cuts or abrasions immediately clean the area with soap and water and apply a antiseptic ointment (like BETADINE or BACTROBAN ointment). You can cover the area with a clean bandage. Do not use kerchief, lungi or sari piece as a bandage as they are not sterile and may contain bacteria. Inspect the injuries next day. If there are any signs of infection like redness, swelling, and pain or any fluid oozing out, immediately consult your doctor.

Avoid exercising for at least one hour after food and do not take food immediately after exercise. Also, do not take cold bath immediately after exercise. Exercising in air-conditioned atmosphere is not advisable. Choose an area with natural ventilation.

How hard should you exercise?

Roughly, you should exercise till you feel tired but not very tired. As I said earlier, go slow in the beginning and gradually increase the intensity of exercise. There is a scientific way of knowing how hard you should exercise. All of us know that our heart beats faster when we exercise. There is something called maximum heart rate (MHR) for different ages. The maximum heart rate (MHR) for a given person can be calculated by subtracting a person's age from 220. One should try to exercise to such an intensity so as to achieve 75% of the MHR, lasting 15 minutes every day and 5-6 days a week (at least 3 times a week). Suppose your age is 50 years. Now your MHR is 220-50=170. 75% of 170 is 127 beats. Hence, you should exercise till your heart rate reaches 127 beats per minute if your age is 50. A heart rate of 100-140 is O.K. as a rough guide. If you have some heart disease, then do not aim for 75% of your MHR. However, you can safely exercise to achieve 40-45% of MHR even with heart disease.

You can check the heart rate by counting the beats at the wrist, neck, or chest for one minute (or counting for 15 seconds and multiplying by 4).

Are you fit for exercise?

Read the following questionnaire carefully and answer each question. If your answer is yes to any question, then talk with your doctor before starting exercises.

1. Do you have a heart problem?
2. Do you experience chest pain at rest or while doing physical activity?
3. Do you often feel faint or have spells of severe dizziness?
4. Do you have any joint or bone problem?
5. Do you have high blood pressure?
6. Did you have any major operation in the last 6 months?
7. Did you have any major injury or fracture in the last 6 months?
8. Are you pregnant?

9. Are you 60 years of age or older?
10. Do you know of any other reason not mentioned here because of which you should not exercise?

When you should not exercise?

There are some situations during which doing exercise is not advisable or may be harmful to you. These are as follows.

Very high blood glucose (> 300 mg/dl with type 1 diabetes, and > 400 mg/dl with type 2 diabetes).

Exercising when blood glucose is very high makes the blood glucose go even higher. This happens due to release of so many hormones in the body during exercise. First, get your blood sugar at least below the above levels by other means like diet, medicines etc and then start exercising.

Low blood sugar

You should not do exercise when your blood sugar is low i.e. less than 80, because it can drop to lower levels. If your blood sugar is low, eat a snack and then start your exercise.

Very high blood pressure (BP)

Exercising when blood pressure is very high can push the blood pressure still higher temporarily. Get your BP under reasonable control and then proceed with exercise. Then exercise can help you in bringing down your blood pressure.

Presence of ketone bodies in the blood or urine (ketosis)

This has been explained in the chapter "complications of uncontrolled diabetes and how to prevent them". Avoid exercise if ketone bodies are present, otherwise it gets aggravated, and may lead to a serious condition called DKA.

Severe proliferative retinopathy.

It is a eye condition in which there are many abnormal blood vessels in the retina of the eye. These abnormal blood vessels may rupture during exercise due to increased blood circulation and BP. Your doctor can tell you whether you have retinopathy or not after examining your eyes. However, minimal retinopathy does not lead to problems when you exercise.

Severe nerve damage (neuropathy)

Patients with severe nerve damage should avoid heavy exercises especially those involving legs. Since there is decreased pain sensation, such people may injure their feet or develop pressure sores.

When you are sick

Exercising during an illness (like fever, cold, diarrhea etc) can delay your recovery or cause the illness to worsen. Rest is required during an illness.

Extremely hot or cold conditions

Exercising in extreme weather conditions is not good for anyone. Your chances of having hypoglycemia (low blood sugar) and dehydration increase in hot weather. Exposure to extremely cold weather can cause frost bite, cracked skin and impaired circulation. When the weather is very cold exercise indoors.

Spondylitis of neck, painful arthritis, recent fractures of bones or recent major surgery.

Any form of strenuous exercise should be avoided. Minor physical activities are O.K. Consult your doctor about your fitness to do exercise.

Warming up and cooling

Do not straight away start doing heavy exercises or physical activity. Warm up for five minutes and then slowly increase the intensity of your exercise to the targeted heart rate. Again, at the end of exercise have five minutes of cooling off period, during which the intensity of the exercise is gradually decreased.

Warming up helps in many ways. It makes your body warmer so that it becomes ready for more exercise. Warming up increases the blood supply to your muscles and makes your body more flexible for further exercise. This flexibility helps you increase the range of motion of your joints and prevents injuries such as muscle tears and pulls. Your heart takes the load slowly without any problem. You can warm up by walking for 3 to 5 minutes and then by doing few stretching exercise. You can also do some simple hand exercises or slow jogging to warm up. To warm up the chest and shoulder area, do a few shoulder rolls, arm circles etc.

Cooling off makes you recover gently. It helps in slowly returning your heartbeat and breathing to normal levels. It takes 3 to 5 min for the body to cool down and come to resting state. A safe cool down period is at least 3 minutes, preferably 4-5 minutes. You may experience dizziness or a "worn out" feeling, if you stop the exercise suddenly without a proper cool down.

One more important thing is, if for any reason your exercise is interrupted, then when you restart the exercise do not restart from where you stopped. You need to warm up again and start with low intensity exercises as if you are starting fresh.

Tips for being regular with your exercise program

Being regular with your exercise program can sometimes be difficult because it requires time, efforts and discipline. The following tips will help you to be regular with your exercise program and continue to gain the benefits from it:

- Choose exercises, which you like. For example if you like swimming, make it your main exercise. It is difficult to continue with something that you do not like.
- Choose a variety of exercises, so that you don't get bored.
- Choose an exercise program, which suits your lifestyle. You are more likely to continue with an exercise program, which does not interrupt your normal life.
- Set realistic goals for your exercise program. By setting unrealistic goals, you become disappointed and may not continue with your exercise program.
- Consistency is the key to creating a new habit. Do your exercise daily so that it becomes a natural habit for you.
- Try to find friends who are engaged in similar activities. Working together is more enjoyable than working alone. For example if you like morning walk try to find some friends who also go for morning walk.

Always remember the following points

- Choose a physical activity that you like and is appropriate for your current fitness level.
- Exercise most of the days in a week (at least 5 days in a week). Aim for at least 30 minutes of aerobic exercise. If you miss 2 or 3 days in a week, it does not matter. However, try to be regular most of the days.
- Monitor blood glucose levels by home testing before and after exercise.
- Carry a food that contains fast-acting carbohydrate in case blood glucose levels get too low during or after exercise.
- Wear or carry a diabetes identification bracelet or card when you go out for exercise.
- Drink extra fluids that do not contain sugar before, during and after exercise.

7 Managing Diabetes with Oral Medicines

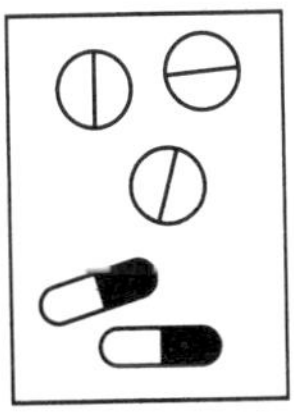

When you are detected to have diabetes for the first time, if your blood sugar levels are not very high, you are most likely to be put on a diet and exercise program. Diet and exercise may bring under control mildly elevated blood sugars and this control may remain for a long time. However, if your blood sugars are very high, or diet and exercise program alone is unable to bring your sugars under control, then you need to take some oral diabetes medicines in addition to diet and exercise. But, note that if you have type 1 diabetes, then oral medicines will not work for you. Type 1 diabetes always requires insulin from the beginning. If you are, type 2 diabetic then oral diabetes medicines will work for you. All the oral medicines that are available can be grouped into 5 categories. These are:

Sulfonylurea Drugs

These are: *Chlorpropamide*, *Glibenclamide*, *Gliclazide*, *Glipizide*, *Glyburide*, and *Glimepiride*.

How they work

These medicines stimulate your pancreas to produce and release more insulin. They work only if your pancreas can still produce some insulin. It is like whipping a tired horse to run fast. Horse can still run but the only thing is it is tired. In the same way in type 2 diabetes pancreas is still producing insulin but not enough. Pancreas needs whipping and that is what exactly these medicines do. If the horse is completely exhausted then whipping will not work. Similarly when the pancreas is completely exhausted and cannot produce any insulin, these medicines do not work. That is why in advanced stages of type 2 diabetes and type 1 diabetes sulfonylurea drugs do not work, because pancreas cannot produce any insulin how much ever you stimulate it.

How often to take

Some sulfonylureas work for full day, so that you need take them only once. Others are taken twice or thrice a day. Your doctor will decide how many times you should take your medicine.

When to take

Take these medicines with food or immediately before food. If you take the medication once a day, you can take it just before breakfast. If you take the medicine twice a day, then take the morning dose before breakfast and the night dose before dinner. Take the medications roughly at the same time each day. Your doctor will tell you when to take your medication, depending on the type of sulfonylureas prescribed.

Side effects

The most common side effect of sulfonylureas is low blood sugar (hypoglycemia), especially in the beginning of treatment till the dose is adjusted properly. If you have liver or kidney problem, then you are at much greater risk of developing low blood sugar because these drugs are neutralized in liver and removed by kidneys. Damage to liver and kidney increases the blood levels of sulfonylurea drugs, which may cause low blood sugar. Glipizide, glyburide, and glimepiride are relatively new and are less likely to cause low blood sugars.

Biguanides

In this group, *Metformin* is the only drug that is being used now.

How they work

We know that liver produces glucose. Metformin works by decreasing the production and release of glucose from your liver. One advantage of metformin is that is tends to cause less weight gain than do other diabetes medications. Another advantage is that metformin does not cause low blood sugars.

How often to take, when to take

Metformin needs to be taken two to three times a day with meals. Metformin now comes in extended release formulations, which means that this medicine gets released slowly in the intestine and hence it works for a long time. Such preparations can be taken once or twice a day. Your doctor will decide about the dose and how many times to take it.

Side effects

Side effects of metformin include a metallic taste in your mouth, decreased hunger (which may be an advantage because it will make you eat less), nausea or vomiting, abdominal bloating, or pain, gas and diarrhea. These effects usually decrease over time and are less likely to occur if you take the medication with food. A rare but serious side effect is lactic acidosis, which results when an acid called lactic acid builds up in your body. Symptoms include tiredness, weakness, muscle aches, dizziness, and drowsiness. Therefore, if you are taking metformin and notice any of the above symptoms consult your doctor. Lactic acidosis is especially likely to occur if you are dehydrated, take alcohol with this medicine, or have kidney damage. Hence, it is not given for people who have kidney damage. Even though metformin has some side effects, it has many advantages and is one of the most common medicines being used for diabetes.

Meglitinides

They include *Repaglinide* and *Metaglinide*

How they work

These medicines work in the same way as sulfonylureas. Meglitinides are less likely to cause low blood sugars than sulfonylureas. They act fast and for short time. They lower blood sugar maximum one hour after taking, and their action gets over in three to four hours.

How often, when to take

You need to take these medicines before meals. If you skip a meal, you should skip the dose before that meal.

Side effects

These medicines can cause low blood sugars and weight gain.

Alpha-glucosidase Inhibitors

These are *Acarbose*, *Volibose* and *Miglitol.*

How they work

We know that the food we eat is broken down in the intestine by enzymes. Glucosidase is one such enzyme present in the intestine, which breaks down carbohydrates into glucose. Alpha-glucosidase-inhibitors block the enzyme glucosidase, hence glucose formation in the intestine is reduced. Unbroken carbohydrate is absorbed slowly from the intestine into the blood, which prevents rapid rise of blood sugar that happens after eating a meal.

How often, when to take

They should be taken with the first bite of a meal. They can be taken one to three times a day. Your doctor will decide how many times you should take. If you skip a meal skip the tablet before that meal.

Side effects

Abdominal bloating, gas, and loose motions. These drugs should mot be used with some newer insulins like lispro and aspart

Thiazolidinediones

These drugs include *Rosiglitazone*, *Troglitazone*, and *Pioglitazone*

How they work

These drugs make your body tissues more sensitive to insulin so that whatever insulin is there it can act more efficiently. They also decrease glucose production from the liver. Both these effects decrease the blood sugar.

How often, when to take

Pioglitazone is usually taken once a day at the same time, with or without a meal. Rosiglitazone is taken either once or twice a day, at the same time each day, with or without a meal. Your doctor will decide about the dose and timings.

Side effects

Side effects include swelling of the body due to water retention, weight gain, and tiredness. A serious potential side effect is liver damage. The thiazolidinedione troglitaone was removed from the market in March 2000 because it caused many cases of liver failure. If you are taking one of these medicines, it's important to have your liver checked every two months during the first year of treatment. Contact your doctor immediately if you experience any of the signs and symptoms of liver damage, such as nausea and vomiting, abdominal pain, dark urine, or yellowing of your skin and eyes (jaundice).

Drug Combinations

Sometimes one medicine may not be able to control your blood sugars. Then using 2, 3, 4 or even 5 medicines together may be able to control your blood sugars. Using 2 or more drugs from the same class will not help. Drugs from different classes have to be combined. Each class of drugs can be combined with drugs from any other class. Most doctors prescribe either a sulfonylurea or metformin first and combine these two if sugars are not controlled by any one of these. More drugs are added if sugars are still uncontrolled. Many drug companies have marketed tablets, which contain 2 or more drugs in a single tablet.

Oral medicines work best when you use them along with diet control and exercise. This way, you have three therapies working together to lower your blood glucose levels.

Can Everyone Take Diabetes Pills?

Diabetes pills don't work for everyone. As I said earlier they do not work in type 1 diabetes. Even in advanced stages of type 2 diabetes some of these pills will not work (sulfonylureas and thiazolidinediones). However metformin and alphaglucosidase inhibitors can work in type 1 and advanced stages of type 2 diabetes. Advanced stage of type 2 diabetes means you have had it for at least last 10 years. Sulfonylureas are unlikely to work in a type 2 diabetic who is taking more than 20 units of insulin per day.

A pregnant woman should not take oral diabetes medicines. She should take insulin throughout pregnancy. This is because oral medicines have many side effects on the baby. But metformin can be used safely in pregnancy.

Diabetes pills may sometimes stop working after a few months or years. When this happens, combining many drugs will help. If even with maximum doses of oral medicines your blood sugar is not controlled, then you require insulin. Insulin can be added to oral medicines. There is no need to stop all oral medicines and take only insulin. Some oral medicines can be continued along with insulin. Best oral medicine to continue with insulin is metformin.

Sometimes when you fall sick, you may need to switch over to insulin temporarily. This is required only if you are seriously ill, have some bad infection, or undergoing some surgery. It is difficult to control blood sugar with oral medicines in such situations. For mild illness and minor surgeries, there is no need to stop oral medicines. If you are very sick consult your doctor and he will decide what to do.

Using Diabetes Pills Wisely

Diabetes medicines, like any other medicines should be used with care. The most important thing that you should remember while using diabetes medicines is low blood sugars. It can happen with most of the diabetes medicines except metformin and alphaglucosidase inhibitors. Whenever you have symptoms of low blood sugar, check your blood sugar with a glucometer or in a lab. If you have many episodes of low blood sugars, consult your doctor because your medicines require adjustment.

Take the medicines at the advised time regularly. It is also important to follow the advise regarding whether medicines should be taken with food. Take your food regularly. Do not skip the meals once you have taken the tablets.

Many diabetes medicines can interact with other medicines. So try not to take any medicines unnecessarily other than the prescribed ones. Whenever you visit a doctor, carry with you the list of all drugs you are taking or still better the drugs themselves.

Some diabetes medicines, which are made long acting by the company, so that you can take them once or twice a day, instead of many times may have special coatings on them. Do not break, crush, or chew before swallowing them. If you do so, their long action may be lost. Each of the drugs mentioned above is manufactured by many drug companies with different names. For example, glimepiride is available as *Blisto*, *Euglim*, *Amaryl*, *Zoryl* etc. These are names given by different companies. Do not change from one brand to another unnecessarily. Stick to one brand unless your doctor tells you to change. There may be quality differences among different brands even if the content is same and there can be differences in their action.

Last but not the least is, once diabetes medicines are started do not think everything is over. Diabetes medicines are started usually at a lower dose and then adjusted as required. So do not forget to visit your doctor frequently, until your blood sugars are under control.

8 Managing Diabetes with Insulin

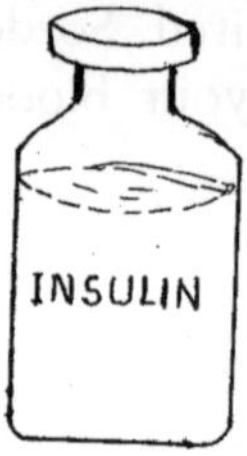

Insulin is a protein hormone produced by the pancreas, an organ that lies in the left side of abdomen. It was discovered by a doctor and a medical student (Banting and Best) in 1920. They got the Nobel Prize for this remarkable discovery. Insulin is necessary for the body to make use of sugar (glucose) to produce energy required by the body. Sugar comes from the food that we eat. All proteins that we eat are digested by us. Since insulin is a protein, it is digested in the stomach if you take it by mouth and it cannot reach blood. Hence, insulin has to be given by injection. However, research is going on to manufacture insulin, which can be taken by mouth.

Currently available insulins can be divided into three groups: animal insulins, human insulin, and insulin analogues.

Animal Insulin

The first successful insulin preparations came from cows (and later pigs). The insulin was isolated from the pancreases of animals slaughtered for food. The bovine (from cow) and porcine (from pig) insulin were then purified, bottled, and sold. Bovine and porcine insulin work well for the vast majority of patients, but some can develop allergic reactions to these animal insulins. These allergic reactions happen because animal insulins are not exactly same as that produced in our body and hence body may think that it is a foreign protein and react against it. Now a days, the use of animal insulin is becoming less and less and many companies have stopped manufacturing animal insulins.

Human Insulin

This insulin is manufactured by genetic engineering techniques. It does not come from people directly but it is same as the insulin produced in our body. Since it is exactly same as the insulin produced in our body, it is more safe and does not produce allergic reactions.

Insulin Analogues

Insulin analogues are recent developments. They are slightly different from human insulin in that one or two amino acids are changed. Such small changes give these newer insulins special properties like faster action or very prolonged action. These newer insulins are lispro, aspart, glargine and detemir.

Insulin is available in many strengths. The most common strengths available are 40 units of insulin per ml and 100 units of insulin per ml. These two are known as U-40 and U-100 insulin respectively. In India, U-40 insulin is the one commonly used. Other strengths of insulin are also available but not commonly used like U-500 insulin. Using U-40 insulin, if you inject 1 ml it is equal to 40 units of insulin. If you have to inject 60 units in one shot then it is better to use U-100 insulin. It is not possible to draw 60 units into the syringe using U-40 insulin, because most of the insulin syringes are of 1 ml capacity only. Therefore, at a time you can draw only 1 ml (40 units) into the syringe. Hence, if you want to inject 60 units you need to take 2 injections. First, you draw 40 units and inject, then again draw 20 units and inject. This is cumbersome and you can avoid two injections by using U-100 insulin. With this, if you want to inject 60 units, you need to draw only 0.6 ml insulin into the syringe. U-500 insulin is used only in people who need to take large amount of insulin.

Insulins can be grouped into 3 categories depending on the duration of action: short-acting, intermediate-acting, and long-acting. Short acting insulins are regular insulin, lispro and aspart. Intermediate acting insulins are lente and NPH insulins. Long acting insulins are glargine and detemir. Short acting insulins control sugar after meals. Intermediate and long acting insulins control fasting blood sugar and provide continuous basal supply of insulin which is necessary for the body even if you don't eat.

Once insulin is injected into the body subcutaneously, it starts acting after sometime (onset of action), produces maximum action after sometime (peak action) and its action lasts for a particular period (duration of action).

Different types of insulins available in the market and their action after subcutaneous injection

Insulin type	*Starts acting in*	*Maximum action*	*Duration of action*
Aspart	5-10 min	1-3 hours	3-5 hours
Lispro	< 15 min	0.5-1.5 hours	3-5 hours
Regular (plain)	30 min	2-4 hours	5-8 hours
NPH/Lente	2-4 hours	4-12 hours	10-18 hours
Ultralente	4-6 hours	6-16 hours	18-20 hours
Glargine	2-4 hours	No peak	24 hours
Detemir	Slow	No peak	Up to 24 hours
Premix insulin (human insulin 30/70)	30 min	Has two peaks.	10-18 hours

Your doctor will tell you what type of insulin you should take, how much to take, and when to take it. It is important to get and use the exact type of insulin your doctor prescribes because different insulins vary in strength and action. Always check the label of the insulin you buy with the doctor's prescription to make sure it is the same.

When do you require insulin?

If you are a type-1 diabetic, tablets will not work for you. Hence, you need to be on insulin lifelong from the time of diagnosis. If you are a type-2 diabetic (which most people are), tablets will work for you. There are many types of tablets available and your doctor will put you on one or two of these tablets initially. However, as type-2 diabetes advances over a period of many years (usually after 10 – 15 years), blood sugar control becomes difficult only with tablets. At this point, your doctor will try to put you on maximum dose of all the available tablets. Even after this, if your sugar is difficult to control, you have reached a point where you require insulin. Most diabetics will reach this point some or the other time. So do not refuse insulin, if your doctor advices you to take it after trying all the available tablets at maximum dose. Sometimes when you are sick, undergoing some surgery, you need to be put on insulin, even if your sugar is well controlled with tablets. After the illness or surgery is over you can be put back on your tablets. Also, a pregnant lady with diabetes requires insulin because tablets cannot be used since they affect the baby.

Storage of Insulin

Insulin should be kept in refrigerator, at a temperature between 2-3°C. It should not be frozen or exposed to higher temperatures.

Discard insulin bottles that have been opened for three or more months, even if kept in refrigerator. Insulin will spoil if it gets exposed to above 90° temperature or if it freezes. Do not leave insulin bottles (or pens) inside a car in hot summer or cold winter. Temperature inside car can go very high in hot summer. If blood sugars rise and there is no other obvious cause, your insulin might have lost its potency especially if it has been opened for more than one month. If for any reason there is a doubt about the potency of insulin, it is better to buy a new bottle.

The solutions of insulin lispro, aspart, regular insulin, glargine and detemir are clear (like water) whereas NPH, lente, and ultralente appear cloudy. Before injection, inspect the vial for any change like clumping, frosting, precipitation, and change in clarity or color. If any of these things are noticed it means that, the insulin is spoilt. If so, do not use the bottle, buy a new one.

Mixing Insulins

Sometimes you need to use two types of insulins to control your blood sugar. In such situations, you need not inject them separately, because this will require two injections. Instead you can mix them together and inject as one shot. Usually these two types of insulins include short acting insulin and intermediate acting insulin. You should know the proper method of mixing insulin. In general, you should draw the short acting insulin first into the syringe and then draw the delayed action preparation. This will avoid contamination of short acting insulin vial with delayed action preparation. Contamination of short acting insulin vial with a delayed action preparation may spoil the short acting insulin vial and make it longer acting. Contamination of delayed-action-preparation vial with short acting insulin does not have any effect on that preparation.

Mixing regular insulin with lente or ultralente insulin (which contain Zn) causes a significant retardation of the onset & peak activity of regular insulin. Hence, it is recommended that neither of these insulins be routinely mixed with regular insulin unless you are already using such a mixture and your blood sugars are well controlled with it.

If you are mixing insulins yourself before injection, you should follow the guidelines below.

- Do not mix any other medication or diluent with any insulin unless told by your doctor.
- Do not mix insulin glargine with any other insulin. This is because glargine solution is acidic and may spoil the action of other insulin.
- Lispro insulin can be mixed with NPH, lente and ultratente. When lispro insulin is mixed with these insulins, the mixture should be injected within 15 minutes before a meal.
- Mixing regular insulin and lente insulin is not recommended except for patients already adequately controlled on such a mixture. If such a mixture is used it should be injected immediately after mixing.

For many people buying two bottles of insulin and mixing them is cumbersome. Hence, many pharmaceutical companies have developed and marketed many premixed insulin preparations of intermediate (NPH) and short acting insulins (regular insulin, lispro and aspart). Mixing short acting with NPH insulin does not change the action of both insulins. Mixtures of regular and NPH are available in the concentrations of 70:30 and 50:50 (70% NPH & 30% regular) (50% NPH & 50% regular). Recently premixed preparations of neutral protamine lispro and lispro, neutral protamine aspart and aspart are also available in the market. Such insulin mix preparations are very convenient to use because you need not go through all those steps of mixing insulins. These preparations have become very popular now and most diabetics who take insulin are on such readymade insulin preparations.

Insulin Syringes

Insulin syringes are available in 0.3, 0.5, 1 and 2-cc capacities. When choosing a syringe, there are four things to consider: which insulin concentration it's designed for, its capacity, the needle size (gauge), and the needle length. Always buy a syringe that's designed for the insulin strength that you use. For example, if you use U-40 insulin, then buy U-40 syringes. If you use U-100 insulin, then buy U-100 syringes; otherwise, you will inject the wrong amount of insulin. Most people use 1-cc syringe. Needle sizes are measured in gauges. The available needle sizes range between 27 and 31 gauges. Higher the gauge, thinner the needle. Thinner the needle, lesser the pain. Use a needle that feels most comfortable for you. Needles come in different lengths, such as 5/16 inch and 1/2 inch. Some insulin pen needles are as short as 1/3 inch. Insulin needles are short to help prevent insulin injections from going in too deeply. Ask your doctor which length needle he or she recommends for you.

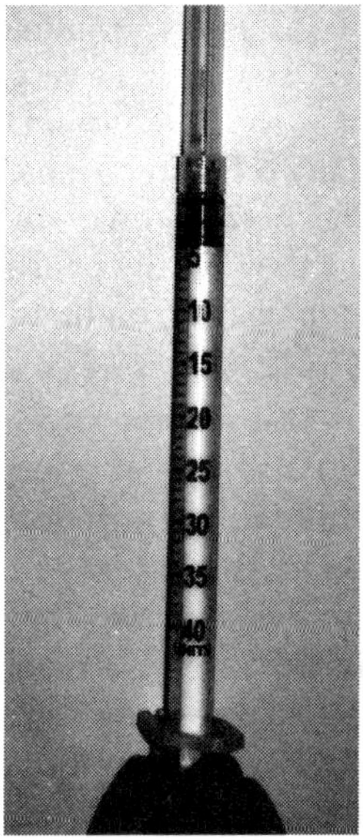

Insulin syringe

Small needles are helpful in young children. Manufacturers of disposable syringes and pen needles recommend a single use. Reuse of syringes or needles carries the risk of infection. However, most insulin preparations have bacteriostatic additives that inhibit the bacteria commonly found on skin. Still some people may be at increased risk of infection. These include persons with poor personal hygiene, and acute concurrent illness, or decreased resistance to infection for any reason. Such persons should not reuse a syringe or pen needle. Some patients find it practical to reuse needles. If needle reuse is planned, it should be recapped after every use. Certainly, a needle should be discarded if it is visibly deformed or dull or if it has come in contact with any surface other than skin. The syringe also may be reused and it can be stored at room temperature. Cleaning the needle with alcohol is not recommended as it may remove the silicon coating on the needle that makes injections less painful. Pen devices though costly, cause less pain and you can carry them with you easily.

How to Inject Insulin

Everyone with diabetes should learn how to inject insulin. Initially it appears scary to inject oneself. Actually, it is very easy and you should do it to see how easy it is to inject insulin. Insulin injection hurts little because unlike many other injections, it is injected into the subcutaneous fat. The needles used for insulin injection are very small and thin that they hardly cause any pain. Most of the needles also have silicon coating on them so they slip easily into the skin.

Of course, even insulin shots can hurt if you do not know how to inject correctly or the needles you use are of poor quality. You should learn the correct technique of injection from your doctor or nurse. Let them observe you when you inject so that they can correct your technique. Even if you think you are an expert in injecting your insulin because you have been doing it for many years, still it is good idea to review your injecting technique from time to time. Without good technique, not only can shots be uncomfortable, but it can also be difficult to attain good diabetes control. The correct technique of insulin injection is as follows:

- Always verify the label before injection.
- Clean the injection site with soap and water or an alcohol swab.
- The insulin vial or pen should be gently rolled in the palm or shaken gently to resuspend the insulin. This is not necessary for short acting insulins, insulin glargine and insulin detemir as they are clear.
- Clean the top of the insulin bottle with an alcohol swab. If you are using a new bottle of insulin, remove the protective cap from the bottle. Do not remove the rubber stopper or metal band under the cap. The rubber stopper keeps the insulin bottle sealed between uses.
- Take your syringe and draw air into the syringe. The amount of air should be roughly same as the insulin dose you wish to withdraw. Now insert the syringe into the bottle and

inject the air into the bottle. Air needs to be injected into the bottle to avoid creating vacuum inside the bottle when you withdraw insulin.

- Draw up the insulin. Turn the bottle upside down (with the syringe still inserted) holding it with one hand. With your other hand, slowly pull back on the plunger to draw the correct dose of insulin into the syringe.
- When mixing short acting with long acting insulin preparations prior to injection, the short acting insulin should be drawn up first in the syringe and then long acting insulin. If you draw long acting first, it may mix with short acting and spoil it.
- After the insulin is drawn, look for air bubbles in the syringe. Without removing the needle from the bottle or changing the position of the syringe or bottle (they should still be upside down and vertical), hold the syringe at eye level. If you see any air bubbles, tap the syringe barrel a few times with your forefinger. This will make the bubbles to float to the top of the syringe. Gently push the plunger to inject the air bubbles back into the insulin bottle. Pull back again on the plunger to redraw your dose of insulin. Repeat this step as needed if you see more bubbles in the syringe. Small air bubbles are not dangerous in themselves, but may decrease the dose of insulin injected.
- Remove the syringe from the bottle. Check the syringe to make sure that you have drawn the correct dose of insulin. The syringe is now ready for injection.
- Injections are given into the subcutaneous tissue. Lift the skin and fat tissue between the thumb and the first finger, and inject at 90° angle, if you are using short needles (5/16 inch) and the fat in the area of injection is adequate. 45° angle can be used for the 1/2 inch needles and for injection in thin individuals and children to avoid intramuscular injection. The needle should be in the subcutaneous tissue for at least 5 seconds if you are using pen device to ensure complete delivery of the insulin dose. It is generally best to push the needle all the way into the skin. If the needle is not in far enough, the insulin may not be injected into the fatty layer. If it goes into the skin rather than into the fatty layer below the skin, it will sting and may cause a small swelling or redness and itching. If the needle is not close to the fingers holding the skin, the gentle pinch can continue to be held during the injection of the insulin.

- Inject the insulin by pushing the plunger down with a SLOW and STEADY push as far as it will go. Some people like to wait a few seconds to let the insulin "spread out" after each five units of insulin is injected. A smooth injection is important. After injecting the insulin, wait 5 to 10 seconds before removing the needle. This will prevent insulin leakage from the injection site. A loss of one drop of insulin may be equal to two to five units. Loss of insulin is a common reason for variations in the blood sugar levels. If "leak-back" continues to be a problem, choose a new site next time. Also, two units of air can be drawn into the syringe after removing the needle from the insulin bottle. Then flick the side of the syringe with a finger to make the air rise up under the plunger. The air will then be injected after the insulin and will help to prevent "leak-back."
- After the injection, place a finger or dry cotton swab over the site of injection. Hold for a few seconds to prevent any bleeding. Rub the site gently to close the needle track. Some bleeding may occur after the needle is pulled out; this is not harmful, although some insulin may be carried out with the blood. Press dry cotton firmly on the site. A clean finger also can be gently pressed over the site where the needle came out and rub the site gently. If an injection seems especially painful or if the blood or clear fluid is seen after withdrawing the needle, apply firm pressure for 5 to 8 seconds at the site without rubbing. Check blood glucose more frequently on the day when this happens. If it is suspected that a significant portion of insulin dose was not injected, check blood glucose within a few hours of the injection.

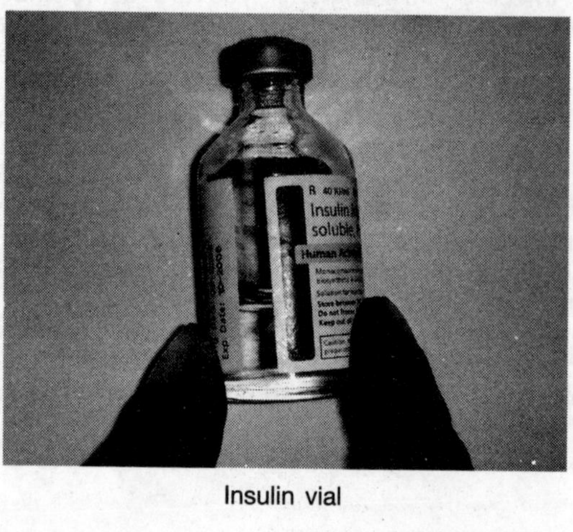

Insulin vial

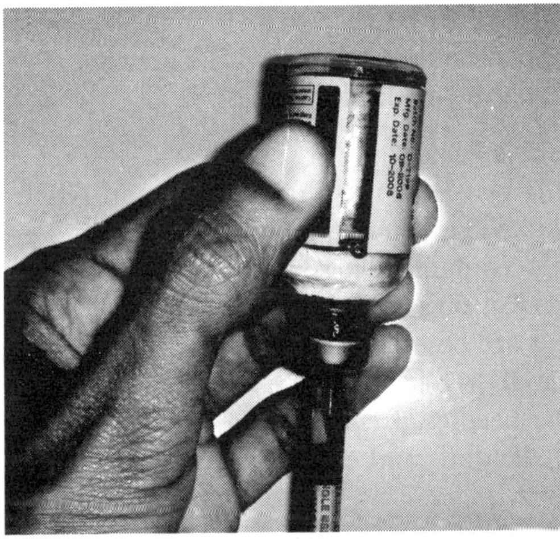

Drawing insulin into the syringe

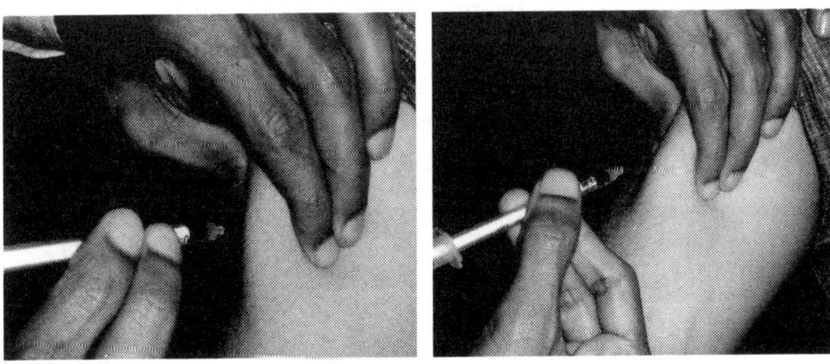

Injecting insulin at vertically (90 degree) and 45 degrees angle

Pen devices for insulin injections

Pen devices are instruments used to inject insulin. They look exactly like the pens that we use to write and can be kept in our pockets. Insulin, needle, and injector are all incorporated into this small pen like instrument. Because insulin pens are so convenient and easy to carry, many people are switching over to insulin pens. The required dose of insulin is dialed & the plunger is depressed after placing the needle in subcutaneous tissue. Insulin pens may be disposable or reusable. In disposable pens, the container inside the pen that contains insulin (called cartridge) cannot be replaced when insulin gets over and the entire pen has to be disposed. In reusable pens the cartridge inside the pen can be replaced with a new one. Insulin cartridges are available in medical stores.

1. Disposable Pens

Disposable pens for lispro, aspart, human NPH, premixed 30/70 Regular/NPH, detemir, premixed lispro, and premixed aspart are readily available. These pens have to be discarded after the insulin gets over. They cannot be refilled. The pens are simple to use and are compatible with small BD 31 gauge (5/16 inch) Ultra-Fine III® needle or a NovoFine® 30 gauge (1/3 inch) disposable needles. Reuse of pen needles is not recommended as the needle dulls and can cause tissue damage at the injection site.

2. Reusable Pens (Cartridge Pens)

These pen devices can be reused after replacing the cartridge. Cartridges are nothing but insulin refills. Cartridges (replaceable) contain usually 1.5 ml (150 units) or 3 ml (300 units) of insulin and can be replaced when the cartridge is empty. You can inject up to 70 units in one shot using pen device.

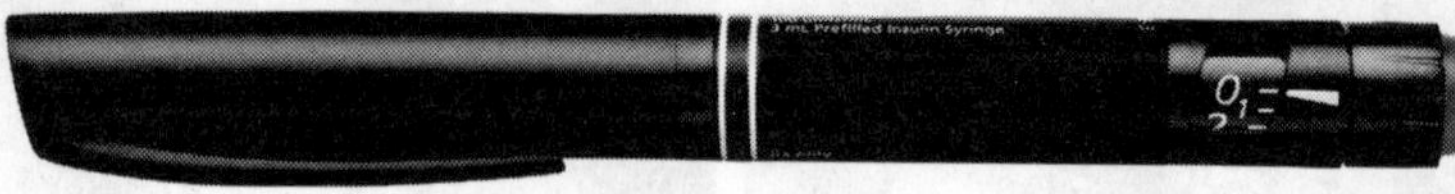

Pen device

How to inject using insulin pen

It is same as injecting with syringe. However, it is more convenient because you need not draw insulin, remove air bubbles etc as you do with a syringe. All that you have to do is,

- Fix a needle to your pen. Follow the directions that come with your pen for fixing a needle. Do not leave the needles attached to pen in between injections. This allows air to enter into the bottle and contaminates insulin. Insulin may also leak out through the needle.
- Roll the insulin pen between the palms of your hands or tip it back and forth at least 15 - 20 times to mix the insulin. Now dial the required dose and inject as you would inject using a syringe.

Once in a while, check whether the pen is working by dialing and discarding 2 – 3 units of insulin. If insulin comes out through the needle then you know that the pen is working. If no insulin comes out, then repeat this again. If insulin still does not come out of the needle, your pen may be empty, needle may be blocked, or the needle may not be connected properly.

Read the instruction manual that comes with your pen. It contains lot of information on how to maintain and use your insulin pen correctly.

Tips to lessen pain while injecting insulin

Insulin injection hardly causes any pain. Here are some tips to minimize the pain.

- Injection of cold insulin causes pain. Hence, take the vial out of refrigerator well in advance of injection, and allow it to come to room temperature and then inject. You can also keep the insulin vial or pen at room temperature for at least 1 month without loss of potency.
- Remove all air bubbles before injection as injecting air bubbles also causes pain.
- Injecting through alcohol causes burning pain, hence, wait until the alcohol (spirit) that you have applied on the skin evaporates completely and then inject.
- Pain can also be lessened by keeping muscles at the injection site relaxed while injecting.
- Penetrate the skin quickly, and do not change direction of the needle while inserting or withdrawing.
- Do not reuse needles. Old, blunt needles cause pain.

Needle blockage

Occasionally, a small piece of fat or the insulin (particularly Ultralente insulin) can plug the end of the needle during the injection. Sometimes it is possible to pull out the needle a little and then push the needle back into a slightly different place. If you still cannot push down the plunger to finish the injection, you have to use a new syringe. Note very precisely the units of insulin remaining in the blocked syringe. Fill a new syringe with the required insulin dose and inject into another site. Needle blockage is not seen with insulin glargine and detemir as they are clear and do not have any suspended particles. If possible, the syringes should be stored with the needle pointing upward or lying flat, so that suspended insulin particles do not collect in the needle and block it.

Jet injectors

Jet injector devices work by delivering a fine (0.008 inch) high velocity stream of insulin into the subcutaneous tissue under high pressure. They are almost painless and are especially useful in children. Jet injectors are not in common use and are yet to become popular.

Where to inject insulin?

Insulin may be injected into the subcutaneous tissue of the upper arm, front and sides of thighs, buttocks and abdomen (with the exception of a circle with a 2 inch radius around the umbilicus). [see Fig. 8.1]

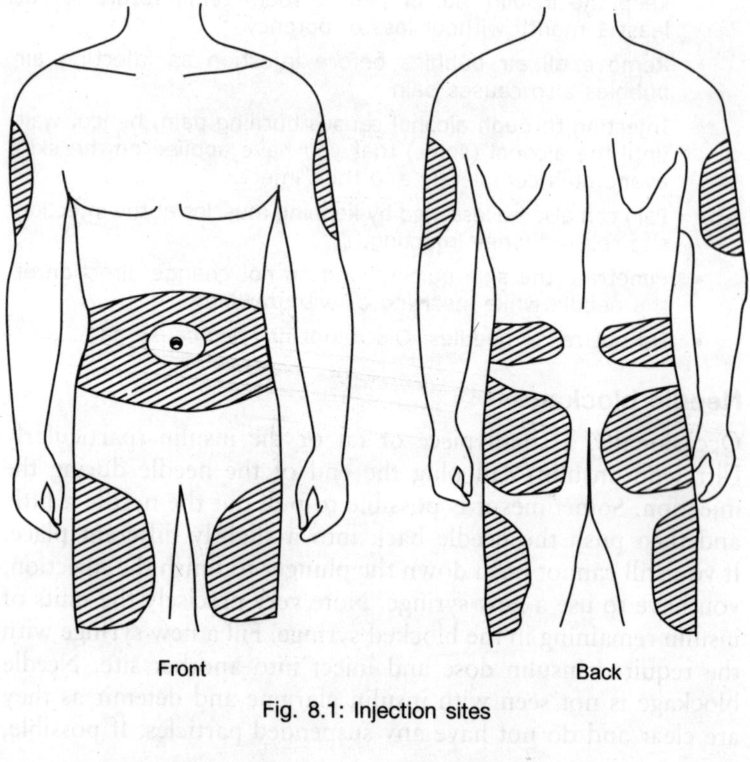

Fig. 8.1: Injection sites

Rotation of the injection sites

Rotation of injection site means injecting into different site each time. I.e. try to avoid the same site for next injection. You need not go to some other area in order to change the site of injection. Rotating within one area is recommended. E.g. as shown in Fig. 8.2 first few injections are rotated in the right arm. Then switch the site to left arm etc. Rotating within one area rather than switching to different area each time will decrease variability of absorption from injection to injection. Rotation of the injection site also prevents the development of lipohypertrophy or lipoatrophy (lipohypertrophy or lipoatrophy means areas where fat becomes very thick or very thin respectively).

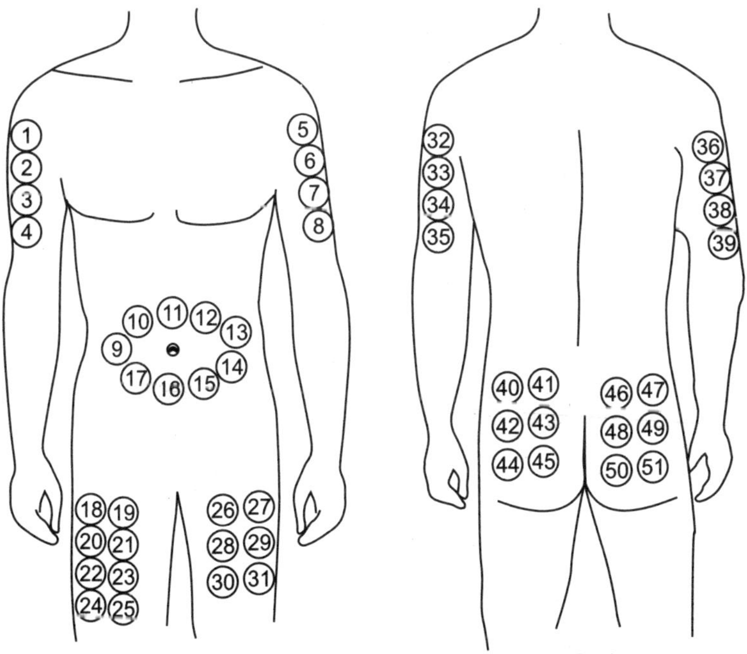

Fig. 8.2: Rotation of injection sites

When to inject insulin?

Some time gap should be given between insulin injection and meals. This is because insulin takes some time to act after injection. After meals your blood sugar level reaches maximum after 1-2 hours. After insulin injection, insulin also reaches maximum level after sometime. This maximum level of insulin should match with the maximum level of blood sugar. This matching is achieved by giving some gap between insulin injection and meals. How much gap to give depends on what type of insulin you are using. For human insulin, which is the most common type of insulin being used, you have to give a gap of 20-30 minutes. So do not start eating immediately after insulin injection, wait for 20-30 min and then eat. There are some new insulin preparations available now (insulin lispro and insulin aspart) which can be injected immediately before a meal or with the meal or even after a meal.

Avoid taking warm shower or bath or getting into a hot tub after taking insulin injection as this increases the blood supply to skin and results in faster rate of absorption which may result in hypoglycemia.

What to do if the injection goes into muscle instead of subcutaneous tissue?

In a person who is very thin or very muscular, there may be little fat under the skin. Injections may go into the underlying muscle, causing more rapid absorption of insulin and low blood sugar. Injections into the muscle are most likely to occur if the syringe is held at 90° angle to the body (unless short needles are used). Sometimes extra pain will occur when injections go into muscle, but this is not always the case. So do not rely on only pain. Check your blood glucose more frequently if you suspect that insulin has been injected into the muscle. If injecting into muscle is a problem, it may be necessary to pull the skin away from the muscle and insert the needle into the "tent" below while still holding the pinch of skin. Since the entire pinch is not being held, just the upper tip, the insulin should not leak-back.

9 Monitoring Your Blood Sugars

This chapter will teach you how often you have to check your blood sugars and how to keep track of your blood sugar levels. Monitoring blood sugar simply means checking it frequently. By checking blood sugar frequently you can know whether it is high or low and treatment can be adjusted according to blood sugar levels. Always remember that adjusting your medicines is an ongoing process whether it is oral drugs or insulin. It is not that you start treatment and forget about it for many months. So many things can push your blood sugar out of control. It may be progression of diabetes, stress, changes in your health, changes in your food, changes in your activity etc. Hence, you need to check your blood sugar frequently. Now a days checking blood sugar has become very easy with the availability of glucometers. You can check your blood sugar yourself at home using glucometer. This process of testing your blood sugar yourself at home is called self-monitoring of blood glucose or "SMBG." It is recommended that all diabetes patients use SMBG to,

(a) Keep track of glucose levels
(b) Help make day-to-day decisions for managing blood sugar
(c) Recognize emergency situations

Laboratory blood glucose tests

Most people check their blood sugar in labs. Testing in lab is the most accurate method of measuring blood sugar. Whenever you visit your doctor for blood sugar check up, he will check blood sugar either by using glucometer or in a lab. Check your blood sugar at least once a month in a reliable lab. Other times you can use glucometer (a small portable instrument) to test your blood sugar yourself. Remember the following points whenever you go for blood sugar check.

- Do not skip any tablets or insulin. Take your usual dose and go. Many people skip medicines or insulin dose and then go for blood sugar check, which is wrong because this will show falsely high values of sugar.
- Test both FBS and PPBS because one can be normal and other can be abnormal.
- To test FBS (fasting blood sugar), give morning blood sample. Do not eat or drink anything in the morning except plain water. The previous night you should have your usual dinner.
- To test PPBS (postprandial blood sugar), have your usual meal. Do not eat more or less than usual. Go for testing 2 hours after the meal. For example if you had lunch at 1 pm, go for testing at 3 pm. You can do PPBS 2 hours after breakfast and dinner also.

Is it OK to test urine sugar to assess diabetes control?

No, not at all. Urine sugar testing to assess sugar control was common earlier because of non-availability of labs and also the cost involved. But now a days almost all the labs do blood sugar testing or you yourself can check your blood sugar using glucometer. Testing urine sugar is not recommended for monitoring blood sugar control, because there are so many things, which can change urine sugar levels. Presence of sugar in the urine is known by urine color change when urine is heated with a chemical called Benedict's reagent. Urine without sugar becomes blue colored when heated along with this reagent. Presence of increasing amounts of sugar makes the urine turn into green, yellow, orange, or red color. Red color indicates that the blood sugar is very high. Urine color change can happen whenever there is protein in the urine. Certain vitamins like vitamin-C also interfere with urine sugar testing. Moreover, urine sugar testing cannot give you the exact blood sugar value; it can only give a rough indication of blood sugar value. For example, urine sugar testing will show red color at 300 mg/dl blood sugar and any value above this, i.e. whether blood sugar is 300 or 600, still urine will show red color. If the blood sugar value is less than 180 mg/dl, urine sugar testing will show blue color. Again here, whether the value is 100 (normal sugar) or less than 50 (low blood sugar), still the urine sugar test will show blue color. Hence, one cannot differentiate between low blood sugar value and normal blood sugar using urine sugar testing.

Because of all these disadvantages, urine sugar testing is not recommended for monitoring diabetes and adjusting treatment. Best thing is to get blood sugar tested at a lab or do it on your own using glucometer.

What is glucometer?

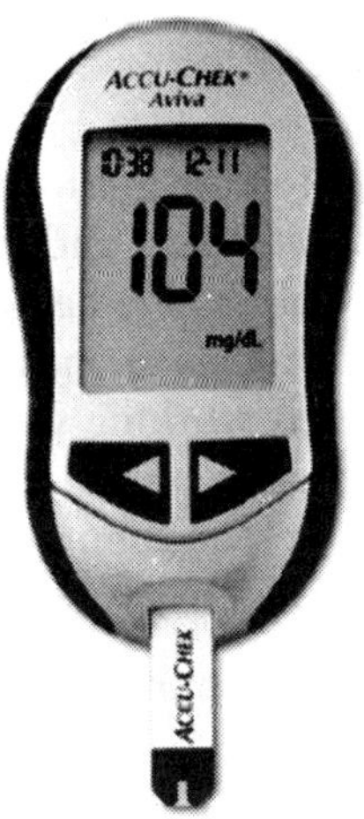

Glucometer is a small portable instrument used to test glucose. Glucometer is just the size of a mobile phone and you can easily carry it in your pocket. Along with glucometer you need test strips to test your blood glucose. Test strips are nothing but paper pieces coated with chemicals (glucose oxidase, dehydrogenase, or hexokinase) that combine with glucose in blood and change the color of the blood. The meter measures how much glucose is present in the blood and displays it as a number. Glucometers can record and store a number of test results. Some models can connect to personal computers to store test results or print them out.

The availability of glucometers has revolutionized the management of diabetes. Every hospital has many glucometers and every diabetic should buy a glucometer. Currently, the market for blood glucose meters is several billions dollars per year worldwide and the sales are expected to increase further.

How to test your blood glucose level using glucometer.

It is very easy! You can learn how to use glucometer from the place where you buy it, or from your doctor, nurse or diabetes educator. You can also attend some diabetes education programmes where they may show you how to use glucometer.

You can also try to learn it by reading the user manual provided with the glucometer. Instructions to test your blood glucose are as follows:

1. Wash hands with soap and warm water and dry completely or clean the area with alcohol and dry completely.
2. Prick the fingertip with a lancet. Lancet is a needle like device available in medical or surgical stores.
3. Hold the hand down and squeeze the finger until a drop of blood appears; apply the drop on the test strip.
4. Insert the test strip into the glucometer.
5. After a few seconds, glucometer will show the blood sugar value. Record the test result.

Take your glucometer with you at least once to your doctor or nurse and test your blood glucose in front of him. Your doctor can watch your technique to make sure you are using the meter correctly. Testing the blood sugar at a lab and by using your glucometer simultaneously can tell you whether both the readings are matching. If they match then it means your technique is correct and your glucometer is working well. Note that there will be some difference between lab and glucometer readings. So do not expect to get an equal number from both. Only thing is there should not be too much difference.

How often should you check your blood sugar?

It is difficult to make a rule about how many times you should check your blood glucose. As a general rule, the American Diabetes Association (ADA) recommends that most patients with diabetes test glucose three or more times per day. Pregnant women taking insulin for gestational diabetes should test two times per day.

Once in while it is better to check you blood sugar before breakfast and after breakfast, before lunch and after lunch, before dinner and after dinner, and at bedtime, i.e. 7 times a day. Everyday you need not check 7 times. But it is recommended that you check 7 times at least once a week. Every day you can check at least fasting blood sugar and 2-hour postprandial blood sugar (Postprandial means after meals). Another option is check your blood sugar each day at different times. In this way, you can know whether your blood sugar is in control throughout the day. You should test more often when you change medications, in unusual stress or ill or have some infection (2-4 hourly). Whatever may be the recommendation, the minimum should be monthly blood sugar testing in a nearby reliable lab.

If your blood sugar is consistently high or low, consult your doctor.

Buying a glucometer

Every diabetic should buy a glucometer. It is cheaper than a cheap mobile phone. There are many glucometer models available in the market. Different models may differ in several ways such as

- Amount of blood needed for test
- Testing speed
- Overall size
- Ability to store test results in memory
- Cost of the meter
- Cost of the test strips used

Important features of glucometers

There are several features of glucometers that you need to understand. These features are often different for different meters. You should understand the features of your own meter.

Measurement Range

Most glucose meters are able to read glucose levels over a broad range of values from as low as 0 to as high as 600 mg/dl. Suppose your blood sugar is 700, since this glucometer measures only up to 600, when you test your blood sugar with this meter, it will show it as high and not 700. Similarly suppose a glucometer lowest range is 25, and your blood sugar value is 10 then the glucometer will show it as low and not 10. You should interpret very high or low values carefully. If you get the glucometer reading as high or low, you should check it again and if the reading is same again, then take immediate measures to correct the high or low reading. For low readings, you can take some sugar-containing snack for immediate purpose. However, the cause of high or low blood sugar has to be found out. So it is better to consult you doctor.

Whole Blood Glucose vs. Plasma Glucose

When you test your blood in the laboratory, they measure the glucose levels in plasma (fluid that remains after blood has clotted). But when you test your blood glucose with glucometer, it measures blood glucose in the whole blood. There is a small difference between lab and glucometer measurements. Plasma glucose is generally 10-15% higher than whole blood glucose (this difference is even more after eating). There are many meters on the market now that give results as "plasma equivalent". This allows patients to compare lab and glucometer measurements easily. It is important for you and your doctor to know whether your meter gives its results as "whole blood equivalent" or "plasma equivalent."

Factors that affect glucometer readings

The accuracy of your test results depends partly on the quality of your meter and test strips and your training. Make sure the test strip you use is compatible with your glucose meter. If you are not sure whether a certain test strip will work with your meter, contact the manufacturer of your glucose meter. Humidity and heat may damage the test strips and affect the blood glucose reading. Also, note that your glucometer reading is not as accurate as lab blood glucose measurement. Glucometer reading will vary by 15-20% of the blood glucose value.

Maintaining your glucometer

Cleaning

You need to keep your glucometer clean. You can clean it with wet soft cloth. But do not immerse it in water. Do not use alcohol (unless recommended in the instructions), cleansers with ammonia, glass cleaners, or abrasive cleaners.

Quality control checks

You should regularly perform quality-control checks according to manufacturer's instructions to make sure that your glucometer is accurate and reliable. Otherwise, it may show wrong values and if you rely on these wrong values, your blood sugar may go out of control. Many things can reduce the accuracy of your meter even though it may appear to work well. There are two ways of doing this quality control check. One is by using *Test Quality Control Solutions*. Another is by using *Electronic Controls*. Test quality control solutions are nothing but solutions with known glucose values. Instead of putting your blood on the test strip, you put the quality control solution and check the glucometer reading. The reading should be same as the glucose value in the solution. If the glucometer reading is different from the test solution value then your glucometer is not accurate and you have to contact the manufacturer of your glucometer for advice. Detailed instructions to do this usually accompany the solution. Manufacturers sometimes include quality control solution with their meter. Otherwise, you can order it separately from a manufacturer or pharmacy.

In the electronic control method, you place a cartridge or a special "control" test strip in the meter and a signal will appear which indicates whether the meter is working properly or not.

New glucometers which do not require finger prick

Researchers are exploring new technologies for glucose testing without finger pricks. One such glucometer is based on near-infrared spectroscopy. This glucometer measures glucose by shining a beam of infrared light on the skin. Since there is no finger prick, it is painless. Lot of research is still going on on these glucometers. At present, they are not in widespread use. These glucometers should not be used as a replacement to standard glucometers. They are used to obtain additional glucose values between fingerstick tests.

Testing for glycated hemoglobin (HbA1c)

It is also known as Glycosylated Hemoglobin. We all know that there is hemoglobin in our blood. This hemoglobin is present inside red blood cells. Red blood cells live an average of 120 days. Sugar is also present in the blood. Some amount of sugar gets attached to hemoglobin which is present inside the RBCs. This is what is known as glycosylated hemoglobin. Normally glycosylated hemoglobin should be less than 7%. When there is high sugar level in the blood, there is more attachment to hemoglobin and hence the level of glycosylated hemoglobin rises in the blood. This happens over a period of 120 days (3 months) because the RBCs live that many days. Therefore, when you measure your glycosylated hemoglobin, you can find out your level of blood glucose, averaged over the last 3 months. Doctors have been using glycosylated hemoglobin test for patients with diabetes since 1976. The test is now widely used in the routine monitoring of patients with diabetes mellitus. One measurement of blood sugar may go high because of so many reasons like stress, illness, extra food etc. But if your glycosylated hemoglobin is normal it means your blood sugar has been under control at least for the last 3 months. In the same way suppose one measurement of your blood sugar is normal but your HbA1c is high (more than 7), it means that your sugars were not under control for the last 3 months.

Get your glycosylated hemoglobin tested every 3 months. If your blood sugar is under good control then it is enough if you check it once in 6 months. If your blood glucose level is kept under good control, your HbA1c level also should be normal since HbA1c value reflects average blood glucose levels of last 3 months.

10 Keeping Your Blood Pressure and Cholesterol under Control

In addition to sugar control, there are some other important things you need to take care of. These include your blood pressure, and cholesterol. Many diabetics have high blood pressure and high cholesterol. All three, i.e. high sugar, high BP and high cholesterol form a "deadly trio" and start hunting you down. Hence, in addition to blood sugar, you also need to keep your BP and cholesterol under control.

Blood Pressure (BP)

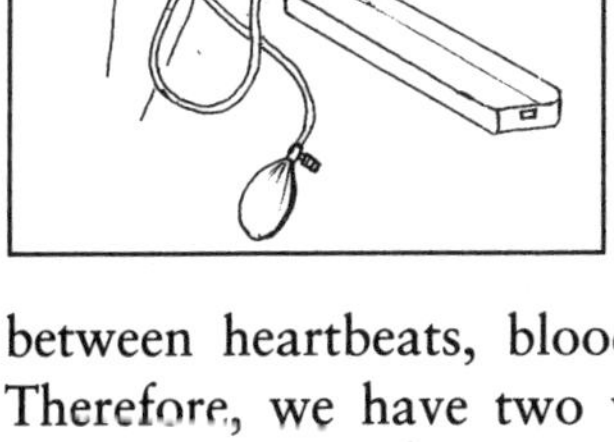

You may be surprised to know that our heart pumps blood more than 100,000 times a day! This pumping creates a pressure inside blood vessels because of which blood flows to all parts of the body. This is like the pressure inside water pipes, which makes the water flow. Each time it pumps blood into the blood vessels, BP rises to upper value. In between heartbeats, blood pressure drops to a lower value. Therefore, we have two values, an upper value and a lower value. Upper value is called systolic BP and lower value is called diastolic BP. That is why blood pressure is recorded as two numbers, e.g., 120/80. Value above the bar (120) is called systolic BP and the value below the bar (80) is called diastolic BP. Both values are important. Even if any one value is high, you have high BP. Normal BP is around 120/80 mmHg. If your BP is always equal to or more than 140/90 mmHg, then you have high BP and you require treatment. Diabetes along with high BP can form a "deadly duo". Both will damage your eyes, kidneys, heart, blood vessels and increase the risk of heart attack and stroke. Both together can do more damage than each one of them does.

Keeping blood pressure under good control is very important for all diabetics. Usually your doctor will check your BP whenever you visit him. A diabetic person has two times more risk of having high blood pressure than a person who does not have diabetes. Hence, it is even more reason for you to check your BP regularly. Most people who have high BP do not have any complaints and only come to know of it very late when they visit their doctor for some other problem. The only way to know whether you have high BP is to get it checked regularly by your doctor. You are more likely to have high BP if you are a diabetic, not active, over 30 years of age, overweight, using too much alcohol and your close family member has high BP. Women who take birth control pills may develop high BP and they should get their BP checked regularly.

How to keep your BP under control?

There are many important things, which you should follow to keep your BP under control.

- Lose weight if you are overweight.
- Cultivate positive emotions like love and sympathy towards others. Say no to negative emotions like anger, hatred, jealousy etc.
- Stop smoking and drinking alcohol.
- Cut down salt intake. High salt intake can increase your BP.
- Cut down oily and fat foods.
- Eat more of vegetarian foods rather than non-veg.
- Do regular exercise, yoga and meditation.
- Get regular medical check ups.
- Take BP medicines regularly as advised by your doctor.

If you adopt a healthy lifestyle, you can cure your BP even without medicines. Lifestyle changes include losing weight if you are overweight, reducing salt intake, reducing fat intake, doing regular exercise, stopping all bad habits like smoking and drinking alcohol. Taking more of vegetarian diet and less of non-veg also helps in reducing BP. Relaxation methods like yoga and meditation also help in controlling high BP. Note that these lifestyle changes also help control your diabetes and its complications.

If lifestyle changes alone are not able to bring down your BP, your doctor will prescribe medicines to control BP. You should continue your healthy lifestyle and also take BP medicines. There are many BP medicines available now and your doctor will decide what medicines are good for you. The choice of medicines will depend on how high your BP is, side effects, presence of other medical problems, and other medicines you may be taking.

Do not take any BP medicine unless prescribed by your doctor. Do not adjust the medicine yourself. Many people wrongly think that whenever they have a headache, it is due to high BP and take extra BP tablet. This is wrong and should not be done. Most of the time headache is due to some other reason. Many people stop taking BP medicine when their BP comes under control, which is also wrong. BP cannot be cured with a course of BP medicines like infections can be cured with a course of antibiotics. BP can only be controlled and it remains controlled as long as you take the medicines. If you stop medicines within a few days, BP again rises.

Finally visit your doctor regularly and get your BP checked. Medicines may need to be adjusted according to your BP.

If you follow all the above things rest assured that your BP will remain under control and you can avoid all the complications associated with high BP.

Cholesterol

If you have diabetes, you have a high risk of developing blocks in blood vessels. When the blood vessels in the heart get blocked you may develop an heart attack. When the blood vessels in brain get blocked you may develop a stroke. These blocks are mainly due to cholesterol deposition. Cholesterol is a type of fat present in your blood. It is present in oils, animal fats, egg etc. You need to check your cholesterol levels in the blood to know whether it is normal or high. This test is called lipid profile in medical language. It is usually done in the morning on empty stomach; hence, it is also known as fasting lipid profile (FLP). Cholesterol test shows your total cholesterol, total triglycerides, high-density lipoproteins (HDLs) and low-density cholesterol (LDL cholesterol). Out of these, HDL cholesterol is your friend because higher the level in your blood, lower is the risk of blocks. LDL cholesterol is known as bad cholesterol because this is the one, which is responsible for blood vessel blocks. The recommended LDL-cholesterol for a diabetic is less than 100. Therefore, if your cholesterol is more than 100, it means you have high cholesterol and you require treatment for this.

How to keep your cholesterol under control?

Healthy diet

Healthy diet can reduce your cholesterol level. Cut down on fats, oils, fried foods, non-veg. Non-veg food is rich in cholesterol. So cut down non-veg and eat more of vegetables. Meat can be divided as white meat and red meat. White meat is white in colour and is also called as lean meat because of its low fat content. Eg- chicken, fish and sea food. Red meat appears red and has high fat content. Eg- mutton, beef, pork, organ meat like liver, kidney. Because of its low fat content, white meat is preferred but even this should not be more than twice a week preferably.

Use less oil for cooking

Cooking methods like steaming, baking or roasting should be used rather than frying in oil to reduce the oil consumption during cooking.

Regular exercise

Helps in reducing blood sugar as well as cholesterol. It also keeps you more fit.

Quit bad habits like smoking and drinking

Both can increase your cholesterol levels and also join hands with cholesterol to damage your blood vessels, kidneys and heart.

Take diabetes and anti cholesterol medicines regularly

There are medicines available to reduce cholesterol level called statins. If your doctor prescribes you one of these, take it regularly. Taking diabetes medicines regularly and keeping your blood sugar under control can also reduce your cholesterol levels.

Now, you know that you have to take care of your cholesterol & BP also. If your diabetes, BP, and cholesterol remain uncontrolled, they form a "deadly trio". If you manage them wisely, a happy and healthy life is yours.

11 Taking Care of your Feet

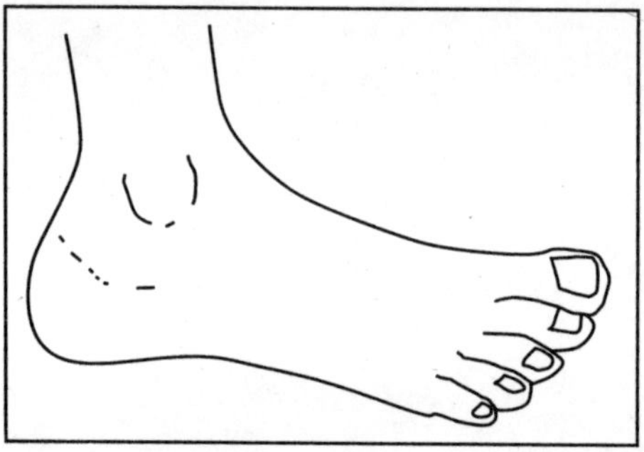

Fig. 11.1: Foot

People with diabetes can develop foot problems. This happens because of many reasons. There may be decreased blood supply to feet in diabetics due to blocked blood vessels. High blood sugar itself leads to poor wound healing and more chances of infection. Another cause of foot problems is nerve damage. Diabetics usually develop nerve damage if sugars are not controlled properly. Nerve damage leads to decreased sensation in the feet and small injuries go unnoticed. These small injuries can become big due to poor healing. Infection and decreased blood supply sometimes may become so severe as to cause gangrene. Gangrene means a dead part and it needs to be removed. A badly infected toe or foot may have to be removed even if there is no gangrene to prevent sepsis. In fact, most of the amputations that are done by surgeons are on people with diabetes. Diabetic foot complications are a major reason for hospital admissions.

However, do not get scared after reading this. Foot problems happen in people whose sugars are uncontrolled and are careless about their feet. That does not mean you should not take care of your feet if your sugars are well controlled. Foot problems are largely preventable with due care. Learn to treat your feet with respect. There are some basic things that you can do to prevent foot problems which have been explained below:

A simple test to know whether your feet are at risk of developing injuries.

Did you know that pain is your friend? Let me give you one example. Suppose you accidentally step on a thorn. Immediately you withdraw your foot from the thorn and try to remove the thorn. Now if you did not have the pain sensation, you would not have felt the thorn prick and would have continued to walk on it. This would have caused damage to your foot. Therefore, pain sensation is the one, which protected your foot from further damage, and hence it is actually your friend. Many diabetics have nerve damage because of which they lose the normal sensations which increases the chances of injuries. There are pressure points on the soles of your feet, which bear your weight on standing (see the Figs. 11.2 and 11.3).

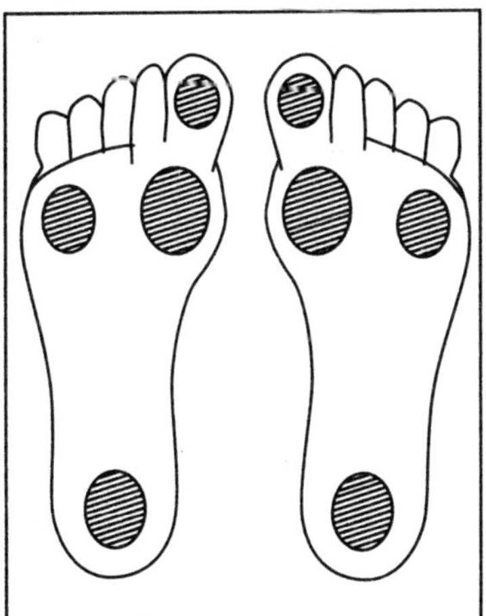

Fig. 11.2: Pressure points on soles

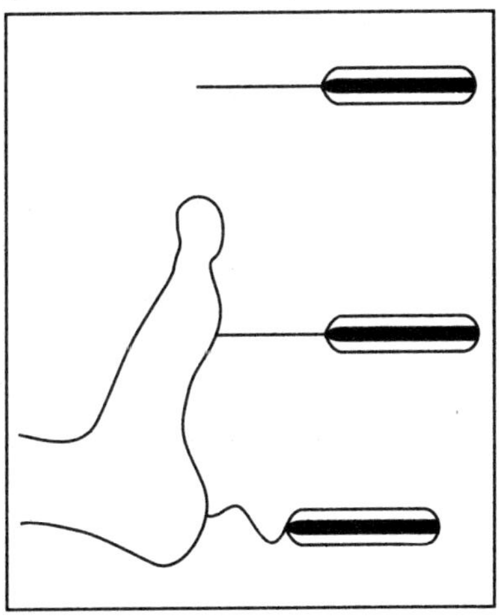

Fig 11.3: Testing touch and pressure sensation with monofilament

These pressure points are the ones, which may develop damage and turn into ulcers especially if you have decreased or absent sensation. Here is a simple test to know whether your feet have normal sensation or not. Buy a 10 gm monofilament which is available in medical or surgical stores (see the figure).

Touch the pressure points on your feet with the monofilament (or ask somebody else to do it) without bending it. If you feel the touch of monofilament, it is normal. Now press the monofilament against the sole until it bends. Now you are checking the pressure sensation (pressure of 10 gms). If you cannot feel the touch or pressure sensation, it means that you have nerve damage and you are at risk of developing foot problems. But all foot problems are largely preventable.

Tips to prevent foot problems

1. Keep your blood sugar under control. This is the first step to prevent all the problems including foot problems.
2. Wash your feet every day with lukewarm (not hot) water and mild soap. Dry your feet well, after washing especially between the toes. Use a soft towel to dry and pat gently. Do not use rough towel or rub hard because it may cuase skin damage through which bacteria and fungus can enter and cause serious infections. You can use powder before putting on shoes, socks, or stockings.
3. Check your feet every day. Use a mirror if required to look at the bottoms of your feet. If you find any open cuts or abrasions clean them with water, apply an antiseptic cream (BETADINE or SOFRAMYCIN skin ointment), and keep the wound covered with clean bandage or BANDAID until it scabs over moist skin. Do not peel the scab. Call your doctor at the very first sign of redness, swelling, pain, or blackish discoloration. Redness, swelling, and pain indicate infection. Blackish discoloration indicates gangrene.
4. Prevent cracks from developing in your feet. Cracks usually develop in winter season. Pathogens can enter through these cracks and cause infection. Keep the skin of your feet smooth by applying moisturizing cream or lotion, especially on the heels. If the skin is deeply cracked, consult your doctor.
5. Take extreme care while cutting your toenails. You should not injure your toes. Even a small injury can get infected and lead to sepsis and gangrene. The best time to cut toenails is after bathing. After a bath, nails are softer and easier to cut. Try to cut the nail straight across, and do not

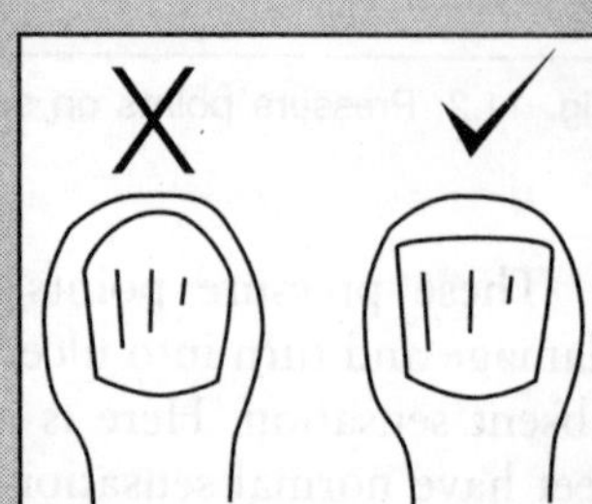

cut the sides of nail. By cutting the sides, you are most likely to injure your toes.

6. While trying to remove the dirt, never probe down the sides of your nail with sharp objects, you may cause a puncture, which can get infected. Pile the corners gently without injuring the skin.
7. Be careful not to burn your feet in hot water or on hot water bottles, near radiators or open fires. Many diabetics underestimate the temperature of water because of decreased thermal sensation. They do not feel the heat of hot water and hence, may burn themselves with too hot water while taking bath. Use warm water to take bath or ask others to check the temperature of water. It is also important to protect your feet from very cold temperature. Best way to do this is to wear warm socks and cover your feet in winter.
8. Wear comfortable shoes and socks. They should not be too tight or too loose. Do not wear shoes without socks. Always wear shoes with soft, comfortable, and clean socks. Wear socks or stockings that are 1/2 inch longer than your longest toe. Do not wear stretch socks, nylon socks, socks with an elastic band or garter at the top, or socks with inside seams. Never walk barefoot. Be careful when wearing a new chappal or shoe because in the beginning they may cause skin injury due to friction. In the beginning, wear your new footwear only for half to one hour every day for many days. Once you get used to your new footwear, then you can wear them throughout the day. Avoid wearing sandals or other open-toed shoes because by chance, if you slip on something you may hurt your toes, which can develop into a bad infection. Also, avoid high-heeled shoes and shoes with pointed toes because they are not comfortable and cause uneven pressure distribution. It is good idea to buy chappals and shoes in the evening, because, in the evening your feet may swell a bit and if the shoes fit you comfortably in the evening they should be comfortable the whole day. Change socks every day. Look inside your shoes every day for things like gravel or torn linings. These things can rub against your feet and cause blisters or sores, which can get infected. If you have any sores or ulcers on the feet consult your doctor. There are special padded shoes and chappals made of microcellular rubber for people with ulcers on the feet.
9. If you have any hard skin or callus on your foot, do not cut it using blade or any sharp object. Corns and calluses may be left alone if not causing any problem. Be careful about

using corn remedies that are available in the medical stores. Most of them contain acids, which can burn your normal skin and cause problems. Use emollient cream for hard skin. Consult your doctor for any problem.

10. If you notice any redness, swelling, pain, or blackish discoloration in the feet or toes, immediately consult your doctor.

Athlete's foot

Athlete's foot is a fungal infection that causes itching, cracking, and redness between the toes or on the soles of the feet. Cracks can get infected and lead to major foot problems. You need to get it treated as early as possible. Antifungal creams can be applied twice a day to treat athlete's foot. It is a better to meet your doctor to make sure that it is athlete's foot and not something else. To use an antifungal cream (CANDID skin ointment), wash your feet and dry well between your toes and on the bottoms of your feet. Rub the cream gently on the affected areas twice a day.

12 What to do during Sickness

A diabetic person can fall ill just like any other person. Some illnesses can be avoided by cultivating healthy lifestyle but you cannot avoid all. A diabetic needs to take more care during illness than a nondiabetic person. This is because the disease fighting ability in a diabetic person may be less. Even seemingly minor illnesses can turn into serious illnesses and pose danger to your life. When a diabetic person is sick, many complications can develop like hypoglycemia, DKA (diabetic keto acidosis), and sepsis.

When you are ill, the first thing to remember is, do not stop your medicines. Many people think that they need less tablets or less insulin during illness because they are eating less. Actually, blood sugar may become high during illness because illness is also a stress and any stress causes an increase in blood sugar. Hence, you should not skip your diabetes tablets or insulin during illness if you are eating normally. Sometimes more insulin may be needed during illness even if you are eating less. Rarely a diabetic person may develop low blood sugars due to vomiting or loose motions if the same dose of diabetes medicines or insulin as before is taken, but most of the time if you have a minor illness, you can safely continue your diabetes medicines or insulin unless you are not able to eat at all.

The best way to know about the status of your blood sugars during an illness is to check it often. You need to check your blood sugar at least 4 times daily during illness. More times, the better it is. By this, you will know whether your blood sugars are going out of control i.e. high or low and you can take corrective actions.

Another important thing is, try to take adequate food and drink lot of fluids during illness. If you are unable to take solid food, and blood glucose is < 180 mg/dl, you can drink sugar-containing liquids like juices, tender coconut water, sherbet, soft drinks etc to provide energy to the body. Note that your body needs glucose to produce energy and fight illness. In fact, low glucose in the blood is more dangerous than high glucose in the blood.

Insulin and illness

Do not straightaway skip your insulin when you are sick. Even if you are not able to eat, you require insulin especially the basal insulin. If you are able to eat normally, you may even require extra dose of insulin. You should never skip your basal dose of insulin. Normally the body requires a continuous basal supply of insulin (basal insulin) whether you eat or not. If you eat, body requires extra insulin to cover the meals (bolus insulin). Therefore, even if you are not able to eat you require the basal dose of insulin. For this, you should know what these basal insulins are. Basal insulins are NPH, lente, glargine and detemir. If you are taking one of these, continue it even if you are not able to eat. Bolus insulins are regular insulin, lispro and aspart. You can skip these insulins if you are not able to eat. If you are taking a mixed preparation where basal and bolus insulins are mixed (e.g. *Human Mixtard, Huminsulin-30/70, Insugen-30/70*), you need to reduce or increase insulin depending on your blood sugar. In any case, never skip insulin, even the bolus insulin without checking blood sugar. If you are unable to check your blood sugar, then you can skip bolus dose insulin. The best guide is blood sugar level. Check your blood sugar every 4 hours. Anything less than this is a compromise but better than not testing at all. You can do some minor adjustments of insulin at home as told above based on these blood sugar measurements provided you have minor illness or pending doctors visit.

Diabetes Pills and Illness

If you are taking diabetes pills, you must watch for signs of low blood sugar during any illness that causes you to vomit or prevents you from eating and drinking normally. The best way is to keep checking your blood sugar every 4 hours using glucometer or whenever you feel that you are having low blood sugars. If you can eat and drink normally during an illness, then continue taking your pills. Even if you cannot eat normally, you can get enough calories and prevent low blood sugars by eating soup, crackers, or toast, or by drinking fruit juices (with sugar) or cola.

What to eat when you are sick

If you are sick and not able to eat normally, try taking small frequent feeds. Small frequent feeds are better tolerated than large feeds. If you are not able to take solid food, try liquid diet like ganji, juice, coconut water etc. When you are sick, you need to get good hydration and calories. You can get adequate hydration by drinking water or any other drink every half an hour. You can get enough calories by drinking sugar-containing liquids like fruit juices, sherbet, cola, tender coconut water, buttermilk, tea, or coffee with sugar, soups, ganji etc. Try to drink l/2 cup of any of these at a time every half to one hour. If you try to drink a big glass at a time, you may vomit it. Once you are feeling better, try adding soft foods like toast, bread, idly, cooked cereals etc or small amounts of food from your usual meal. Avoid spicy and oily foods.

Note that drinking sugar-containing liquids will do no harm to you; instead, they will provide energy to your body to fight the illness and makes you feel energetic. It will also prevent the body from using fats to produce energy. Burning fat for energy produces ketones, which can be dangerous. Drinking sugar-containing liquids also prevents blood sugar from dropping too low. You need not drink these sugar-containing liquids if you can take your usual food or your blood sugar is very high. Remember that during illness you need to do some balancing act i.e. neither should you allow blood sugar to go high nor should you allow it drop low.

When to visit your doctor?

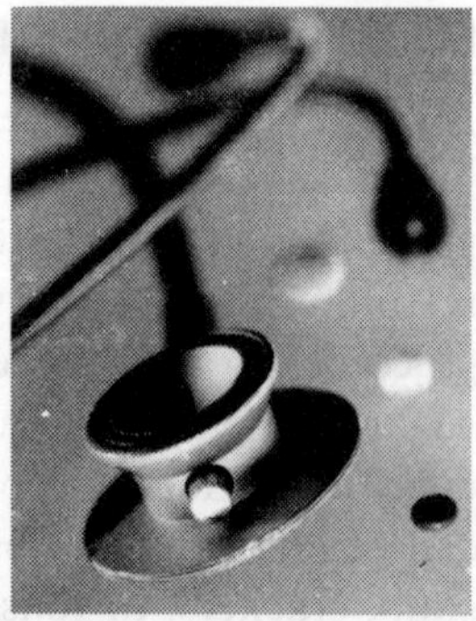

You can try some medicines at home like fever medicines, painkillers, cold remedies etc, but consult your doctor because the nature of your illness has to be diagnosed and treated. Do not assume that every fever is flu and every headache is due to cold. Visit your doctor immediately if you have any of the following:

- Blood sugar level more than 250 mg/dl
- There are ketones in your urine
- Vomiting lasting more than 8 hours
- Loose motions lasting more than 8 hours
- A high or rising fever
- Any illness lasting more than 2 days
- Inability to eat
- Any illness where you feel very weak

13 Low Blood Sugar – How to Recognize and Manage

Blood sugar can sometimes fall too low in a diabetic who is taking treatment (insulin or oral pills). Low blood sugar is also called hypoglycemia. When blood sugar falls to less than 70 mg/dl, it is called hypoglycemia. We can expect every diabetic to develop low blood sugar some or the other time. If you cannot recognize hypoglycemia, you may become unconscious and may even lose your life. Hence, it is important to know how to recognize and manage hypoglycemia. Most of the episodes of hypoglycemia can be prevented if you know why hypoglycemia develops. There are many reasons for hypoglycemia, which have been explained below.

Causes of low blood sugar (hypoglycemia)

Excess dose of insulin or tablets

If you by mistake take extra dose of insulin or tablets, then you may develop hypoglycemia. This is common in old people with poor eyesight. Since they cannot see properly, extra dose of insulin may be drawn and injected. Try to be careful about the dose of insulin or tablets. Make sure that you have bought the correct strength of tablets or insulin from medical store.

Eating less food than usual

Being a diabetic, your food should be consistent from day to day. Being consistent means, eating the same quantity of food every day regularly at the same time. Little variation is O.K., but there should not be too much variation. Your diabetes pills and insulin may have been adjusted to your usual diet. If you suddenly eat less quantity while continuing to take same dose of medicines, then you may develop low blood sugars. If low blood sugars are due to this reason, then there is no need to change the dosage of your insulin or pills. All that you have to do is, be more consistent with your food. If you plan to eat less at any time plan beforehand and try to decrease the insulin dose by 2-4 units or take less medicine that day before the meal.

Missed or Late Meals

This also can cause low blood sugars if you are on insulin and/or oral diabetes pills. Once you have taken your insulin or tablets, they continue to act and missing a meal will produce low blood sugars. You need to be very careful, if you are not able to eat after taking insulin or tablets. Check your blood sugar often. Try to drink some sugar containing drink such as fruit juice, coconut water, or cola to avoid hypoglycemia. You can also eat sweets to prevent hypoglycemia. So try to be more regular with your meals. If you want to skip a meal, then reduce the dose of insulin before that meal. If you are taking short acting insulin before every meal, then if you skip a meal you have to skip the insulin before that meal. Similarly, taking insulin or tablets at the usual times, but eating late can also cause low blood sugars. One situation where this can happen is functions and parties, where there can be delay in serving or having food. The best way to avoid this is planning ahead. Carry your insulin or tablet with you and take them when you are sure that food is going to come within half-an-hour.

Alcohol intake

Taking alcohol can make you eat less food and stimulate insulin release, which can cause hypoglycemia. Alcohol can cause low blood sugars even in people without diabetes. Alcohol can also cause dehydration and lead to an attack of DKA or lactic acidosis. It is wise to avoid alcohol if you are a diabetic, especially drinking too much in one sitting.

Extra physical activity

Your diabetes medicines and food being the same, if you do some unusual physical activity, it can lead to low blood sugars. Extra physical activity means requirement of extra calories for which sugar gets used and blood sugar level drops down. So try to be consistent with your physical activity. Doing too much activity on one day and doing little another day is not good. It becomes difficult to adjust your medicines and blood sugars go up and down.

Problems at the injection site

The sites into which you inject insulin daily may develop some changes over a period. These changes include thinning or thickening of fat at the site (lipoatrophy and lipohypertrophy). Thinning of fat may lead to increased absorption of insulin, which may cause low blood sugars. The best way to avoid such skin changes is to rotate injection sites. I.e. avoid injecting into same site every time. Keep changing the site. This has been explained in the chapter on insulin with diagrams. Read that chapter for more details on injection site rotation.

How to recognize low blood sugars?

There are many signs and symptoms, which can signal that you are having low blood sugars. If you are aware of these, you can detect hypoglycemia early and take corrective measures. If blood sugars become very low, you may become confused, drowsy or you may even lose consciousness. That time you may require the help of a friend or relative to help you treat your hypoglycemic episode. If you are unconscious, you may need to be taken to hospital.

Trembling

Trembling is a common early symptom of hypoglycemia. Initially you may notice very subtle trembling, which others cannot observe. When trembling becomes more, others can also notice it. Trembling is noticed most commonly in the hands because of which you may have difficulty performing tasks such as writing, buttoning your shirt, holding a cup or glass etc. If you are not using your hands, however, you may not notice any trembling. Your tongue also can tremble and your speech can become altered.

Sweating

Sweating is another common symptom of hypoglycemia. Sweating occurs all over the body—not just in the armpits. Many people notice it first on the face. Sweating may be so profuse, that it may drench your body fully. So be careful about sweating occurring in unusual situations like while resting, in cold weather etc, it may be due to hypoglycemia. Extra care is needed to recognize abnormal sweating occurring while exercising, in hot weather etc. In such situations, you might not even realize that you are sweating and you may attribute your sweating to exercise and hot weather.

Fast heartbeat

Fast heartbeat can be an indication of low blood sugar. You may feel that it is beating faster and louder. Many things in addition to hypoglycemia can cause a fast heartbeat, including excitement, stress, nervousness, and exercise. However, when there is no apparent reason for fast heartbeat, you should check your blood glucose level.

For some people who take beta-blockers, a type of blood pressure medicine, sweating may be the only early symptom of hypoglycemia, because beta-blockers can prevent the body from shaking or having other hypoglycemia symptoms such as a fast heartbeat.

Looking pale

When you have low sugars, blood supply to skin reduces. Because of this, you appear pale which may be noticed by you or those around you.

Feeling hungry

Excessive hunger may signal that you are having low sugar. Hunger is a useful symptom of hypoglycemia since it makes you eat and corrects low sugar level. However, sometimes you may ignore hunger when you are at work, in a meeting, engrossed in studying, or attending a lecture. If you ignore hunger, your sugar level may further go down and you may become drowsy and unconscious which requires help from others to treat your hypoglycemia.

This is a dangerous habit to have, because the longer you ignore hunger, the hungrier you get and the more likely you are to overeat when you finally eat. In addition, if you wait until you have moderate hypoglycemia, your judgment may be affected such that you eat the first thing you find, whether or not it will quickly raise your blood glucose level.

Weakness and fatigue

These symptoms are directly related to your body not having enough energy (glucose) for both physical and mental needs. It may be tempting to take a nap when you feel weak and tired, but it's important to monitor your blood glucose level if you feel this way at a time of day when you are not usually tired. If hypoglycemia is causing your feeling of fatigue, your blood glucose level may go even lower during your nap, and you are unlikely to be able to detect other symptoms of hypoglycemia while asleep.

Headache

Headache often signals that you are having low blood sugars or had low blood sugar earlier in the day. For example, if you wake up with a headache or leave a movie theater with a headache, you may have been hypoglycemic for some time but you could not notice it because you were asleep or engrossed in movie. Check your blood sugar more times on such days to make sure sugars are O.K. subsequently.

Problems with vision

Double vision and blurred vision may occur when you have low blood sugar. Like headache, impaired vision often signals that your blood glucose has been low for quite some time. Our brain routinely takes two images from two eyes and fuses them into a single image. When our brain does not have enough glucose, the brain cannot fuse the two images into one. Hence, you may see two things instead of one when you are having low blood sugar. You may see fine with one eye closed, but with both eyes open, you may see double. If you are becoming hypoglycemic while reading, you may notice that you cannot find the correct line or that you see fewer words with each glance.

Difficulty in communicating and understanding

You may notice difficulty in understanding what others are saying. You may appear to others as if you are daydreaming or lost in your own thoughts. You may also have difficulty in getting the right words to speak. Your speech may become slurred and you may respond only in simple words such as "yes" or "no."

Without adequate glucose, your brain has trouble taking in new information. If you find yourself reading the same paragraph over and over or listening to someone speak then realizing you missed what was said, perhaps because you were daydreaming, you may have hypoglycemia.

Dizziness

You may feel lightheaded or experience a reeling sensation. You may have trouble walking a straight line or changing body positions. You may appear to others as if you are drunk because you may sway from side to side while walking. It is wise to carry an identification that you are a diabetic with you whenever you travel outside. In emergencies, this will help others to recognize that you are a diabetic and get you the necessary treatment.

Tingling and numbness

Tingling and Numbness in the face or hands may be symptoms of hypoglycemia. Initially it may be noticed in fingers or lips and, then it may be experienced in other parts of the body.

Unusual behavior

Anxious, confused, and irritable behavior may be due to hypoglycemia. It helps if family members and friends are aware of such a possibility. You may not recognize your family members and friends. Sometimes you may start shouting loudly and behave violently. You may not be aware of your unusual behavior. It can be mistaken for a psychiatric problem and you may even be taken to a psychiatrist.

Unconsciousness

This happens in severe hypoglycemia. If a person develops hypoglycemia in sleep, he may not wake up in the morning. If any diabetic is unconscious, hypoglycemia should be suspected. Do not try to feed glucose through mouth when a person is unconscious, he may aspirate. Glucagon injection can be given if one is available. Family members or friends should shift the person as early as possible to hospital.

Hypoglycemia while driving

Hypoglycemia can happen while driving. If it happens while driving, obviously, there are many dangers involved. You may develop dizziness, become drowsy, may not understand what is happening around and unable to judge properly which may lead to an accident. Because of these dangers, some countries have special rules to issue driving license to diabetics, especially those who are on insulin. Sometimes the warning signals of hypoglycemia like hand tremors and sweating may be ignored while driving, because you may attribute hand tremors to steering wheel vibrations and sweating to hot weather.

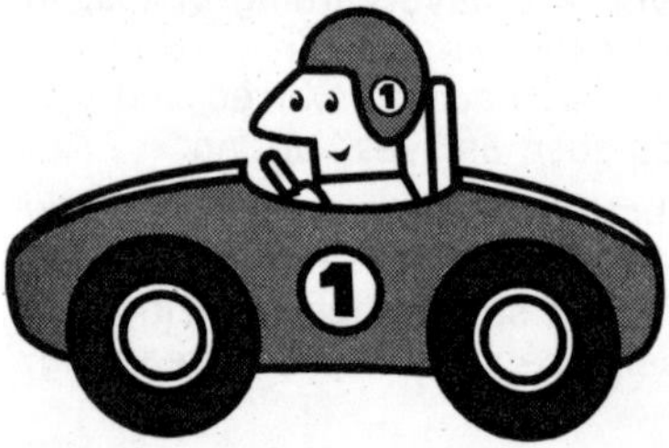

One way to lower your chances of experiencing low blood glucose while driving is to always check your blood glucose level before you start driving. If you are taking a long drive, carry your glucometer with you, stop, and check blood glucose level every two hours. Keep eating some snacks on the way. It is good idea to carry some sweets, chocolates, and snacks with you. Do not delay or skip your meals while driving.

Drivers experiencing hypoglycemia may forget where he is now and to where he is going. Traffic sense may be lost. They may forget familiar roads. They may also forget traffic lights.

Because developing hypoglycemia is dangerous to you as well as to others on the road, you should take all the precautions told above. Whenever you notice any signals of hypoglycemia, do not continue driving. Stop on one side and check your blood glucose with glucometer. If you do not have glucometer, then assume that you have hypoglycemia and immediately take corrective steps like eating sweets, chocolates. Before you start driving, check blood sugar again to make sure, it has returned to normal.

It is good idea to wear or carry some medical identification like bracelet, or booklet showing that you have diabetes with you whenever you move. When you are drowsy, unconscious and cannot help yourself, others may identify that you have diabetes and you may receive the necessary medical help in time.

Wearing or carrying medical identification specifying that you have diabetes is always a good idea, and it's especially true while driving. If you pass out at the wheel or are driving erratically because of hypoglycemia, other drivers and the police may assume that you're drunk. In addition, if your blood glucose level is so low that you do not recognize the authority of the police, you may argue or fight with an officer who pulls you over or approaches you, increasing the likelihood that he'll think you're under the influence of alcohol or other drugs.

However, the police are required to look at a person's wrist, neck, and wallet for medical identification. If you have it, you have a better chance of getting the treatment you need. If you don't have it, you may be placed in a holding room at a jail and not receive any help.

Because others could mistake hypoglycemia for something else, many parents of teenagers with diabetes require that their teens get in the habit of wearing identification before they are allowed to take driver's education. Parents should instruct their teens to check their blood glucose level before driving and delay driving until their blood glucose is in a safe range. These same rules should be followed by drivers of any age who are at risk for hypoglycemia. If you frequently experience severe hypoglycemia, however, you may not receive a physician's clearance for a driver's license until you have proven that your diabetes is under control.

Hypoglycemia while sleeping

If hypoglycemia happens when you are awake, you can recognize it by the above signals. What if you are sleeping? It is difficult to recognize hypoglycemia in sleep. All the signs and symptoms of hypoglycemia like tremors, dizziness, sweating, and fast heartbeat are of no help if you are in sleep. However, there are some symptoms, which may wake you up or partially arouse you from sleep. These include, the following:

Excessive sweating may drench you and makes you feel cold and wet. This may wake you or your spouse. If you wake up and notice that you are sweating and your clothes are wet, do not go back to sleep. Check your blood sugar or eat some sweets and sleep.

Having a headache in the middle of the night or upon waking is a symptom of hypoglycemia. If that happens you should be more careful and check your blood sugars. If you have any doubt, eat some sweets.

Nightmares or strange dreams can be a symptom of hypoglycemia. Some people keep having the same types of dreams during hypoglycemia. Try to recognize how your dreams are different during nighttime hypoglycemia and respond to it by getting up and checking your blood glucose level if you notice such dreams.

Many times nighttime hypoglycemia is recognized by others because you are sweating excessively during sleep, not arousable or having fits. Fits can happen during severe hypoglycemia.

If you notice nighttime hypoglycemia, you should immediately treat it by eating glucose powder, sweets, or drinking some juice. You should also eat a good snack and then only go back to sleep, because you may again have hypoglycemia if you do not eat a snack. You may require medical help if you are unconscious and not arousable or having fits.

After an episode of nighttime hypoglycemia, you should always try to find out the cause, so that you can prevent it from happening again. Is it because you ate less food? Is it because you took extra tablets or insulin? Is it because you did lot of physical activity? If you find any of these causes, you can easily correct them. If you cannot find out the cause or correct the problem on your own, consult your doctor.

Doing minor adjustments in insulin dose when sugar is low.

You can do some minor adjustments in insulin dose yourself if your sugar is repeatedly low until you meet your doctor. However, before that make sure that low blood sugar is not due to less or no food intake or doing excess physical activity. If less food or more exercise is the cause of low sugar, then you should correct the same and not adjust the insulin dose. Minor adjustments are as follows:

If you are on two injections of mixed insulin daily.

Most of the diabetics are on two injections of mixed insulin daily (a mixture of short acting and intermediate action insulin. Most commonly used preparation is human insulin 30/70).

If FBS is less than 80 mg/dl, reduce night dose of insulin by 2 units.

If PPBS is less than 80 mg/dl reduce morning dose of insulin by 2 units.

How to manage low blood sugar?

If you have any one or more of the above signs and symptoms, suspect low blood sugar (hypoglycemia) and take the following steps:

- Immediately check your blood sugar using glucometer if you have one. This will confirm whether you are having low blood sugars or not. If your blood sugar is less than 70 mg/dl, you are having low blood sugar and you should take the steps described next. Even if you do not have a glucometer, then also you should follow the steps anyway.
- Stop what you are doing and act quickly. Take some sugar in a form that is absorbed quickly like glucose-D powder, or a glass of fruit juice, or 3 Dextrose tablets or soft sweets, or two tablespoons of honey or jam or chocolates. This will raise your blood glucose level and you will begin to feel better within 15 minutes. If the symptoms don't subside within 15 minutes, take more sugar and check the sugar level again. Once the symptoms subside, take some food like biscuits or bread, or your next meal if due.
- Very low blood sugar levels can make you drowsy or unconscious. If so, you will need help from others. They

should not give you anything by mouth if you are very drowsy or unconscious. This is because when you are drowsy or unconscious, whatever they give you by mouth cannot be swallowed. There is a danger that it may enter into your lungs, cause chocking, and difficulty in breathing. They should put you in a side position. If one of your family member or friend knows how to give glucagon injection or dextrose injection they should give it to you. You should also call an ambulance if necessary. Recovery should occur within 15 minutes after giving Glucagon (glucogon is an emergency injection, which should be kept by all diabetics at home. Injection can be easily given by any family member once they learn it). After recovering, you should eat some food like biscuits or bread or meals if it is due.

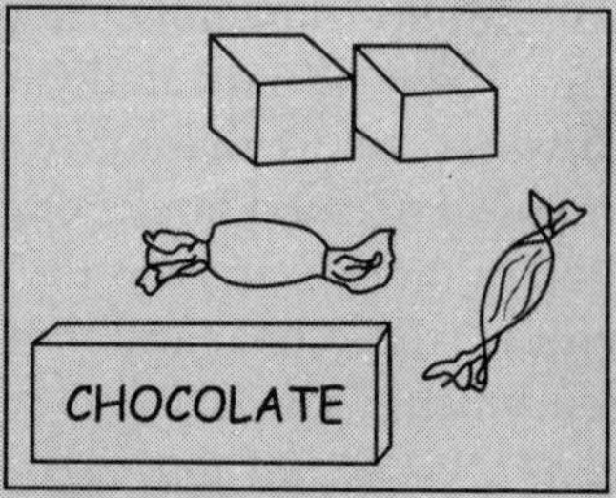

14 High Blood Sugar —What to Do

When you have high blood sugars, there are many things to consider. If you are a newly diagnosed diabetic and just started on treatment, it is usual for your blood sugars to remain high for sometime until the tablets take effect. Even if you are started on insulin, do not expect your blood sugars to become normal within hours. It may take a few days or weeks to adjust your tablets, insulin, or both to bring your blood sugar under control. In emergency situations like emergency surgery, high blood sugars can be brought under control by giving insulin drip. So do not panic if your blood sugars are not under control for a few days or weeks after starting treatment. Attempting fast sugar control by high dose of tablets or insulin may push you into an attack of hypoglycemia. Hence, doctors usually go slow and adjust your treatment slowly.

Maintaining normal blood sugar is a dynamic process. By dynamic process, I mean it is an ongoing process and requires continuous effort. It is not that once your blood sugar is brought under control, you can forget about it and continue to take the same dose of tablets or insulin. Blood sugar may go out of control anytime and there are so many reasons for it. These reasons are,

1. Eating more than usual diet
2. Less than normal physical activity
3. Skipping tablets or insulin or taking less dosage
4. During stress or illness,
5. Natural progression of the disease
6. Some medicines like steroids

Glucose balance in the body

Glucose levels are maintained in the body by a fine balancing act, i.e. balance between factors which increase blood sugar and factors which decrease blood sugar. Food, glucogon and production of glucose by the liver tries to increase blood sugar level and prevents hypoglycemia. Insulin and exercise decrease blood sugar level. Glycogen (which is a storage form of glucose present in liver and muscles) also plays an important role in this balancing act. When there is ample glucose in the bloodstream, the liver converts some of it into glycogen for storage. When the body needs more energy, such as during a prolonged period of fasting or exercise, the liver converts stored glycogen back into glucose so that the body can use it. In emergencies when glucose is not available to the body, it can make use of proteins and fats to produce energy. This can happen in prolonged fasting, where glucose supply from food is cut off. Another situation is enough glucose is there in the body, but the body cannot use it due to insulin shortage. This is what happens in diabetes. There is more glucose in the body, but the body cannot use it because of less insulin or insulin resistance. Hence, body tries to use proteins and fats. Two dangerous complications can happen when blood sugar becomes very high and fats are used to produce energy required by the body. These two are DKA and HHS which have been explained in the chapter 17.

Doing minor adjustments in insulin dose when sugar is high.

If your sugar is not more than 250, you can do some minor adjustments in insulin dose yourself until you meet your doctor. However, before that make sure that high blood sugar is not due to excess food or skipping exercise. If excess food or less exercise is the cause of high sugar, then you should correct the same and not increase insulin dose. Minor adjustments are as follows:

If you are on two injections of mixed insulin daily.

Most of the diabetics are on two injections of mixed insulin daily (a mixture of short acting and intermediate action insulin. Most commonly used preparation is human insulin 30/70).

- If your PPBS is more than 150 but less than 200 increase your morning dose by 1 unit.
- If your PPBS is more than 200 increase your morning dose by 2 units.
- If sugar is more than 250 see your doctor as early as possible.
- If FBS is more than 150 increase the night dose by 1 unit.
- If FBS is more than 200, increase the night dose by 2 units.

Do not increase the insulin dose more than this without consulting your doctor because of risk of hypoglycemia. Do not attempt to adjust tablets yourself.

Actions to be taken when your blood sugar is high

- Whenever you notice a high blood sugar reading (either you have checked yourself with glucometer or in the lab) try to think which of the above is the cause. Next day, try to correct that and recheck your blood sugar. For example if you think eating more food was the cause of high sugars, then next day, eat your normal meals and recheck blood sugar. If blood sugar is still high, you need to contact your doctor to adjust the tablets or insulin.
- Check the expiry date of your tablets and insulin. Expired tablets and insulin lose their action and cannot control blood sugar. Inspect the insulin bottle. If the insulin appears clumpy or there are floating particles in it discard the bottle and buy a new one.
- Whenever your blood sugar is more than 250 mg/dl, check your urine for ketone bodies. This can be done by yourself using KETOSTIX strips or in a lab. If ketone bodies are present, you need to see your doctor urgently, because you may be developing a serious complication known as DKA (diabetic ketoacidosis). If you cannot check ketone bodies, no problem. Meet your doctor, and he will do whatever is necessary.
- See your doctor immediately if your blood sugar is more than 300 mg/dl even if there are no ketones in the urine. As I said earlier, this much high blood sugar can push you into an attack of DKA and HHS. These two dangerous complications may develop when blood sugar goes more than 250 - 300 mg/dl. DKA and HHS can kill a person if not treated in time. Because they can occur in anyone with diabetes, everyone should know what causes them, how to

prevent them, how they are treated, and when to seek medical attention.

- Drink more water and keep yourself well hydrated until your sugars are brought under control. High blood sugar can cause dehydration.
- Do not do any exercise when blood sugar is very high. I.e. more than 300 mg/dl.

15 What Your Family Member or Spouse should Know About You

There are some basic things, which your family members or anyone who stays with you should know. Your family members are also part of your diabetes care team.

First thing is, let all of them know that you have diabetes, especially your spouse. If they know that you have diabetes, they can be helpful in many ways. Obviously, it is very helpful in emergencies. Your family members can help you keep a watch on what you eat, remind you about your medication and sugar testing. Your family members have a great role in altering your eating habits so that you will be eating a healthy diet.

Let all your family members know how to recognize hypoglycemia (low blood sugars). If your hypoglycemia is mild, you can help yourself. However, the problem comes when it is so severe as to make you drowsy or unconscious. When you are very drowsy or unconscious, you are helpless and need help from others. Your spouse or family members can be of great help during such times. If they can recognize that it is due to hypoglycemia, they can take simple measures (like giving you a glucagon injection) to help you come out of it or take you to your doctor.

Let your family members know how to give insulin injections. You yourself can teach them how to inject insulin if you already know how to inject. Although you are the one who is supposed take your insulin injections everyday, sometimes when you are sick or injured and unable to give yourself insulin shots, your family members can give you insulin injections. This way you can avoid multiple trips to hospital or doctor or nurse to take insulin injections. I have seen many people making two to three trips to hospital only because their family members do not know how to give insulin injection.

Another important thing is that they should know how to give glucagon injection, when you have severe hypoglycemia and unable to help yourself. Glucagon is an emergency injection, which will correct hypoglycemia. It can be injected into the muscle or into the subcutaneous tissue just like insulin. All diabetics should buy one injection of glucagon and keep it at home. Let your family members know where you have kept the injection.

Let them know your doctor's and hospital number. Always keep an emergency ambulance number with you and give it to your family too.

16 What You should Always Carry with You

It helps in emergencies if you carry some basic things with you always. Try to carry the following things with you.

An identification which shows that you are a diabetic

Identification can be a bracelet, a small diary, or a card showing that you have diabetes. You can also include other health problems you may be having in this identification. For example hypertension, heart problems or any drug allergy. In case of emergencies where you cannot help yourself (example, when you are unconscious due to hypoglycemia), this identification card helps bystanders or doctors to immediately recognize your problem and give appropriate treatment.

Sugar cubes and chocolates

Always keep some sugar cubes or chocolates in your pocket especially when you go on a long journey. They will be of great help when you unexpectedly develop hypoglycemia. Hypoglycemia can develop anytime in a diabetic and you should be fully prepared to manage it. Eat sugar cube or sweets at the first sign of hypoglycemia even if you are not sure that it is hypoglycemia because it is always better to overtreat hypoglycemia than suffer serious complications.

A glucagon injection and syringe

Carrying a glucagon injection and a syringe to inject it can also save you from suffering a serious attack of hypoglycemia. Carry this injection with you especially when you travel long distances. The advantage of glucagon injection is that, others can inject it to you if you are unconscious due hypoglycemia.

Your medicines and insulin

Carrying your medicines and insulin with you helps you to be regular with your medications. You will not miss any doses if the tablets or insulin is available with you. Many people miss afternoon doses, simply because they do not carry medicines with them. Similarly, when you go for parties and functions, carry your medicines, and take them at the required time. Insulin pens are very convenient to carry in your pocket. It is wise to invest in an insulin pen if you are taking insulin.

Glucometer

If you are going on a long journey or to a far away place, carry your glucometer and glucose testing strips with you.

Glucometers are small in size and easy to carry in your pocket. Check your blood sugar if you experience any hypoglycemia symptoms and take necessary steps to correct it. Also in a remote place, where there is no lab facility to test your blood glucose, glucometer is indispensable.

Your home address and phone number

Keep in your pocket your home address and phone number. It can help others to contact your family members in case of emergencies.

17

Complications of Uncontrolled Diabetes & How to Prevent Them

One of the most common fears that diabetics have is what will happen to them in future. Will they die early? Will they lose their leg or eye? You might have seen hundreds of diabetics who might have gone blind, lost a limb, ended up with kidney failure or heart attack, or developed stroke. All this may be true but what is also true is that there are hundreds of diabetics who do not have any of these complications and are leading a normal life. What makes this difference? It is the blood sugar control that makes the difference. Just go and check any diabetic who has developed a complication. You will find that he has neglected his diabetes. So it is in your hands, get your diabetes under control and you will have very less chances of developing diabetes related complications.

There are many complications, which can happen to you if your blood sugar remains uncontrolled. These can be immediate complications or long-term complications. Immediate complications are DKA and HHS, which can kill a person if not treated in time. Long-term complications are blood vessel blocks, kidney damage, eye damage, heart attacks, stroke, and foot problems.

IMMEDIATE COMPLICATIONS

Diabetic keto acidosis (DKA)

When insulin in the body is absent (as in type 1 diabetes) or there is less insulin in the body (type 2 diabetes), naturally blood glucose becomes high. In spite of this ample glucose in the blood, body cannot use it. Hence, the body uses fat to produce energy. Note that you require energy even if you are resting or sleeping. Because heart has to beat, blood has to circulate, lungs have to breathe, and so many things should go on in the body without interruption. Now, when fats are burnt by the body to produce energy, along with energy something more called ketone bodies are produced. These ketone bodies have acidic properties. So if large amounts of ketone bodies are produced and accumulate in the blood, blood turns acidic. When the blood turns acidic, there are many dangers involved in it. We can survive only if our body maintains a neutral environment. Acidic environment in the body stops the functioning of all the organs. High blood sugar in the body is filtered by kidneys and hence, large amounts of glucose starts appearing in the urine. Glucose in the urine also draws water from the body into the urine. Hence, the person urinates more frequently; the body becomes dehydrated and loses important minerals called *electrolytes*, which include sodium and potassium. Having the proper amount of electrolytes is critical to many body functions, including heartbeat and breathing. If not treated in time, all these serious imbalances can eventually lead to coma and death. This is what is known as diabetic keto acidosis (DKA).

DKA is more likely to happen in type 1 diabetes than in type 2 diabetes because there is no insulin at all in type 1 diabetes whereas there is at least some insulin in type 2 diabetes. Hence, type 1 diabetics should be especially careful about their blood sugar.

HHS (Hyperosmolar Hyperglycemic State)

Hyperosmolar hyperglycemic state (HHS) is same as DKA except that there are no ketone bodies and acidosis in HHS. Like DKA, HHS also happens when there is very high blood sugar and insulin deficiency. As in DKA, people with HHS urinate frequently and become dehydrated. HHS is more likely to happen in type 2 diabetics because they have enough insulin secretion left to prevent the breakdown of fats and subsequent acidosis. Even so, because of the extreme dehydration, HHS can be life threatening and even more difficult to treat than DKA.

Common Triggers for DKA and HHS

Both these conditions can occur in anyone with diabetes, whether he has Type 1 or Type 2 diabetes. However, DKA happens more often in people with Type 1 diabetes and HHS happens more often in people with Type 2 diabetes.

There are many things which can trigger an attack of DKA and HHS. These include,

- High blood sugar: Whatever may be the trigger this is the main cause of DKA and HHS. All other triggers work through high blood sugar levels.
- Inadequate insulin or medicines: Inadequate insulin and medicines may be due to less dosage, skipping insulin or tablets. Sometimes special instruments called insulin pumps are used to deliver insulin continuously to the body. Any malfunction in these insulin pumps may stop insulin delivery and cause insulin deficiency.
- Infections and illness: Any infection can trigger an attack of DKA or HHS. Infections like pneumonia, gastroenteritis, flu are very common. Other illnesses like heart attack, stroke etc can also precipitate an attack of DKA or HHS.
- Any major stress to the body, physical or emotional can increase blood sugar level and cause an attack of DKA or HHS.
- Alcohol abuse: Alcohol can cause dehydration, which can contribute to DKA and HHS.

How to suspect an attack of DKA and HHS

Both DKA and HHS start from high blood sugar. If your blood sugar is more than 250 mg/dl, it is better to check your urine for ketone bodies. Excessive thirst, increased appetite, frequently passing urine, should make you suspect that you are having high blood sugar levels. These symptoms may be present for a few days before DKA and HHS develops. Dehydration is always present in both conditions. Signs of dehydration include dryness of the mouth, cracked lips, sunken eyes, decrease in bodyweight, and flushed dry skin. As the situation worsens, vomiting, weakness, confusion, and coma may occur. DKA may be associated with abdominal pain and vomiting. DKA is also associated with fast and deep breathing. A "fruity" odor may be present in the breath, due to the presence of ketones (acetone). This fruity odor is present only in DKA and not in HHS.

How to prevent DKA and HHS

Prevention is better than cure. Since both DKA and HHS are dangerous and can take away ones life, it is wise to prevent them from developing. For this, follow the tips given below:

- First and most important thing is keep your blood sugars under control. For this check your blood sugar regularly, take your medicines regularly, exercise regularly, and follow diet rules regularly.
- Because infection is a common trigger, beware of any infection and get treatment promptly.
- When you are sick, do not skip your usual doses of insulin or diabetes pills. Of course if you are unable to eat anything, then you may have to reduce your insulin or tablets, but it is not desirable to stop them fully. Best guide is your blood sugar level. Check your blood glucose frequently and adjust the insulin dose accordingly if you can, otherwise consult your doctor. You should also check your urine for ketones when you are sick and if there are ketones you need to be more careful and quick in consulting your doctor.
- Alcohol can cause dehydration, which can contribute to DKA and HHS. Do not drink alcohol in binges. I.e. drinking too much at a time. However, people with well-controlled diabetes can consume alcohol safely in moderation. "Moderation" means no more than two servings of alcohol a day for men and no more than one serving of alcohol a day for women.

Treatment

Both DKA and HHS are dangerous and require emergency treatment. They can kill a person if not treated and require hospital admission for treatment. You will be put in intensive care unit usually. In the hospital, if you are taking oral medicines they will be stopped temporarily. Insulin will be given through intravenous route (directly into the blood vessels) to control your blood sugar. In addition, lots of fluid will be given to you through intravenous route to correct dehydration. If you have any electrolyte imbalance, that also will be corrected. Doctors will also figure out what went wrong and caused DKA or HHS. If infection is the cause, you will be given appropriate antibiotics. If inadequate insulin or medicines is the cause dose will be adjusted. All this may require 2-3 days of hospital admission or even more if there is some serious problem like heart attack, stroke, or serious infection, which might have pushed you into an attack of DKA or HHS.

Lactic acidosis

Lactic acidosis is another diabetes-related crisis worth knowing about. Lactic acidosis is nothing but the accumulation of lactic acid in the body, which turns the blood into acid. It happens especially if you are taking metformin or any drug containing metformin. It is a potentially dangerous condition if not treated in time. Many things can trigger an attack of lactic acidosis. These triggers include dehydration, infections, prolonged exercise, vomiting, excessive alcohol intake, kidney disease, and liver disease. Symptoms of lactic acidosis include lightheadedness, tiredness, weakness, muscle pain, feeling cold, or abdominal pain. If you are on metformin and notice any of the above symptoms consult your doctor. Lactic acidosis is treated by stopping metformin, hydration, and other supportive measures.

LONG-TERM COMPLICATIONS

People who have had diabetes for many years are likely to develop many complications. These complications can be minimized by keeping blood sugar under good control. Long-term complications are:

Blood Vessel Blocks

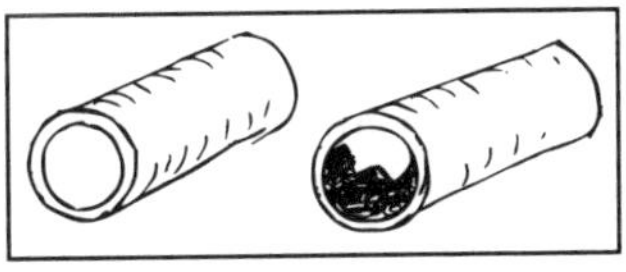

Blood vessels can get blocked very early due to uncontrolled diabetes. High blood sugar damages the blood vessels and cholesterol, which is a type of fat gets collected inside the blood vessels causing these blocks (see the fig showing a normal & a blocked blood vessel). Hence, it is important to keep cholesterol under control in addition to blood sugar. High BP and old age also can lead to blood vessel blocks. Blood vessel blocks can develop anywhere. If they develop in blood vessels supplying blood to the heart, it can result in heart attack (myocardial infarction). If the blocks develop inside the brain, the result is stroke where the person develops weakness on one side of the body (paralysis), speech problems and many other problems. It is a pity to see many relatively young people bedridden due to stroke because of poor diabetes management. If the blocks develop in the legs, gangrene may develop in the feet and feet may have to be removed.

How to prevent blood vessel blocks

- The most important thing is to keep your blood sugar under control. Better the sugar control, the lesser the chances of developing blood vessel blocks.
- Stop smoking. Smoking damages your blood vessels and leads to blocks. Smoking despite of having diabetes is the most dangerous thing you can do. Both will lead to more damage than each one of them can do.
- Cut down fats and oils from your food. Also cut down non-veg. they contain lot of cholesterol. Eat more of vegetables. Take anti cholesterol medicines regularly if your doctor has prescribed them.
- Keep your BP under control. If BP remains uncontrolled for a long time, it can lead to blood vessel blocks. Take your BP medicines regularly if any.
- Become active. Physical activity increases blood circulation and prevents blood vessel blocks.

Heart Attacks

Heart attack is known as myocardial infarction among doctors. Heart attack simply means permanent damage to some part of the heart due to stoppage of blood supply. Because of damage, heart cannot pump the blood properly, which means less blood supply to all parts of the body. A small heart attack may not have much effect on the pumping ability of the heart. However, a severe heart attack damages a significant portion of the heart and affects pumping ability leading to heart failure. A person with severe heart attack may not be able to do much work. He becomes breathless on doing physical activity. A severe heart attack can kill a person. Stoppage of blood supply happens due to blood vessel blocks. As I said earlier, blood vessel blocks can happen due to old age, smoking, high BP, uncontrolled diabetes and high cholesterol. About old age, we cannot do anything because everyone grows old, but other things are in our hand to take care of. Note that uncontrolled diabetes is a major cause of heart attacks.

Stroke

Stroke means an area of the brain suddenly stops functioning. This sudden stoppage of brain function is due to either a blocked blood vessel in the brain leading to absent blood circulation or sometimes rupture of a blood vessel due to high BP. Our brain is a complex supercomputer. Different areas of brain control different parts of the body. Our speech, leg and hand movement are all controlled by different areas of the brain. Also, note that right side of the brain controls left side of the body and left side of the brain controls right side of the body. Whenever any part of the brain is damaged and stops functioning, we cannot move the part controlled by that part of the brain. This is called paralysis. For example, a person with left sided brain damage cannot move right side of the body and also cannot speak properly (speech is controlled by left side of the brain). Diabetics have high chance of developing a stroke due to blood vessel blocks or associated high BP. It is a pity that many diabetics develop stroke and become crippled which could have been prevented if they had managed their diabetes well.

How to prevent heart attacks and stroke

Since the same risk factors lead to both heart attacks and stroke, the following tips will help you to minimize or prevent both.

- Keep your blood sugar under control. This is the most important thing to do to prevent heart attacks and stroke.

- Stop smoking. Smoking damages your blood vessels and leads to blocks, which in turn can lead to heart attacks and stroke.
- Keep your cholesterol under control. High cholesterol causes blood vessel blocks, which in turn leads to heart attacks and stroke. Cut down fats and oils from your food. Also, cut down non-veg because it contains lot of cholesterol. Eat more of vegetables. Take anti cholesterol medicines regularly if your doctor has prescribed them.
- Keep your BP under control. High BP can lead to blood vessel blocks or sometimes cause rupture of blood vessels leading to heart attacks and stroke.
- Become active. Physical activity increases blood circulation and prevents blood vessel blocks.

Eye Damage (Diabetic Retinopathy)

Diabetes is the leading cause of blindness in the world. There are many small blood vessels in the eye which supply retina.

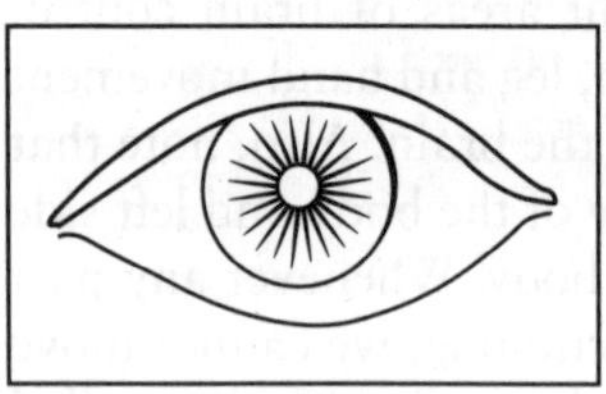

Retina is actually a small screen, which contains numerous small nerves from which a main nerve called optic nerve starts. Retina is very important for normal eyesight. If blood vessels supplying retina get blocked retina develops damage. This is known as diabetic retinopathy. Sometimes the blocked blood vessels may swell up and rupture causing bleeding inside the eye. A person may develop permanent blurring of vision or blindness because of diabetic retinopathy. After 15 years of diabetes, 80% of diabetics will have some diabetic retinopathy. Cataracts (the lens in the eye turns white) are also more likely to develop in diabetics.

How to prevent eye damage and blindness

- Most important thing is to keep your blood sugar under control. All eye diseases and blindness can be prevented or minimized by good sugar control.
- Make it a point to get your eyes checked by an ophthalmologist at least once in a year.

- Do not buy and apply eye drops or ointment on your own whenever you have any eye complaints. Consult your doctor.
- Always wear protective goggles whenever you travel, especially on a two-wheeler. Fast blowing wind and dust can damage your eyes and cause eye infections, which can be prevented by goggles.
- If you have already developed some eye damage (diabetic retinopathy), further damage can be prevented by appropriate treatment. One such treatment is *Laser Treatment* where extra and weak blood vessels in your retina are burnt by *Laser* before they rupture and cause problems. Your doctor will tell about the need for *Laser Treatment*.

Kidney Damage (Diabetic Nephropathy)

Kidneys are one of the main organs in the body. There are two kidneys, one on each side of the backbone inside the abdomen. They appear like kidney beans. Each kidney is about the size of your clenched fist.

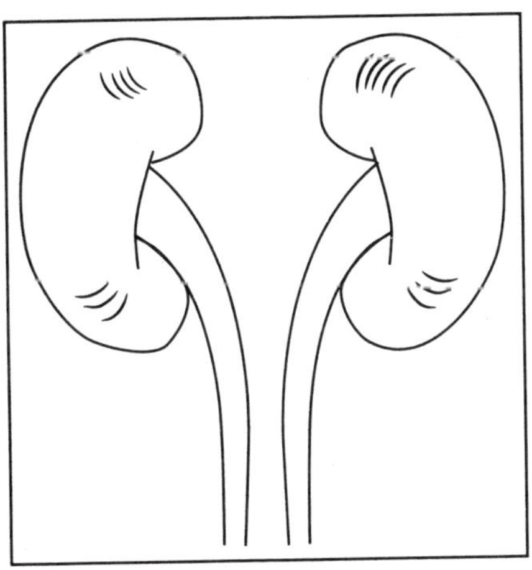

Kidneys do many important jobs in the body but the main job is removing waste products from the body. Two main waste products are urea and creatinine. These waste products are eliminated from the body in urine. Kidneys normally produce one to two liters of urine every day depending on how much fluids we drink.

Whenever there is kidney damage, the levels of urea and creatinine in the blood rise. One kidney can overwork and compensate for the loss of other kidney. Hence, people can donate one kidney without much problem. However, if both kidneys fail, then the waste products in the body have to be removed artificially, otherwise the person will die. This process of artificially removing waste products from the body by filtering blood through a machine is called dialysis.

Kidneys also suffer damage from uncontrolled blood sugars. Most of the kidney failure cases are due to uncontrolled diabetes. It happens because small blood vessels in the kidneys get blocked and result in kidney damage. Diabetes is commonly associated with high BP, which can also result in kidney damage. When there is kidney damage, kidneys cannot filter the blood normally and proteins in the blood can leak into the urine. One such protein is albumin. Albumin starts leaking into the urine very early in kidney damage. Presence of albumin in the urine is called albuminuria. So you need to test your urine for the presence of albumin and its presence indicates early kidney damage. You are lucky if your kidney damage is detected early because there is treatment to prevent further kidney damage. When there is advanced kidney damage, urea, and creatinine (two waste products in the body) which are normally removed by the kidneys start collecting in the blood. So high blood levels of urea and creatinine indicate significant kidney damage. Very late stages of kidney damage require regular dialysis, which may cost any where between 5,000 to 15,000 per month. Another option is kidney transplantation, which may cost lakhs of rupees. Urinary tract infections are also common in diabetics, more severe and may result in kidney damage.

How to prevent kidney damage and kidney failure

- Most important thing is to keep your blood sugar under control. This will prevent kidney damage and kidney failure.
- Get your urine checked for the presence of albumin (microalbuminuria) at least once a year. Presence of albumin in the urine indicates early kidney damage. There are medicines called ACE-inhibitors to prevent further kidney damage. Your doctor will usually put you on these drugs if you have early kidney damage.
- If you have any signs and symptoms of urinary tract infection like burning pain while passing urine; frequent urge to pass urine; passing cloudy or reddish urine; lower abdominal

pain or back pain, do not neglect them. Consult your doctor immediately.

- Do not go on taking pain killer tablets unnecessarily on your own for small aches and pains. Painkillers can cause kidney damage if taken for along time.

Nerve Damage (Diabetic Neuropathy)

People with diabetes may develop temporary or permanent damage to nerves. This is known as diabetic neuropathy. Nerve damage happens if diabetes is poorly controlled. Usually the damage starts 10 to 20 years after the onset of diabetes. You start experiencing symptoms such as numbness, tingling, and burning first in your feet. This will slowly progress to involve whole leg and then hands. There may be decreased sensitivity to heat, cold, and pain. Hence, you may not notice small cuts and abrasions, which become big wounds if neglected. There are chances that you may burn your feet with hot water because you may not feel its heat.

How to prevent nerve damage

- Keep your blood sugar under control.
- Stop smoking.
- Keep your blood pressure and cholesterol under control.
- Eat a nutritious diet, low in fat, rich in vitamins and minerals such as greens and vegetables.

Diabetic Foot Problems

The feet of people with diabetes are very susceptible to infection and injury. There are many reasons for this. Diabetics have blood vessel blocks, nerve damage and easily develop infections. All these lead to foot problems. Many diabetes-related hospital admissions are for foot problems, and many foot and leg amputations are performed on diabetics. In India, diabetes ranks after road traffic accidents as the leading cause of foot and limb amputations. If you want to save your feet, you need to keep your blood sugars under control.

How to prevent foot problems and save yourself from an amputation.

Refer to the chapter "Taking care of your feet" for details.

18 Alternative Treatment for Diabetes Mellitus

Alternative therapies are treatments that are neither widely taught in medical colleges nor widely practiced in hospitals. These include Ayurveda, homeopathy, acupuncture etc.

Ayurveda

Ayurveda is of Indian origin and well known for many centuries. It is becoming popular again. In Ayurveda diabetes is known as *Madhumeha*. The symptoms and treatment of diabetes have been described in detail in ayurvedic texts. Ayurveda as a medical science has penetrated so deeply into the causes and treatments of diseases that no other medical science has such deep insights. Ayurvedic texts have been largely misinterpreted. Ayurveda has suffered a lot due to so many quacks practicing it. Beware of unqualified quacks who destroy both Ayurveda and your health.

What does ayurveda say about diabetes mellitus?

Ayurveda says that diabetes comes due to excess intake of foods with *Madhura* quality and physical inactivity. *Madhura* quality means foods, which are heavy, difficult to digest and have cold properties. Such foods include sweets, rice, wheat, fruits, oils etc. The common belief that eating sweets causes diabetes may have come from this. Ayurveda also says that diabetes develops in persons who are sedentary, sleep excessively, and eat frequently before the previous meal is digested.

Does ayurvedic treatment work?

Remember that ayurvedic treatment is not just administering drugs. There are many things involved in it. You need to correct your eating habits, need to change your lifestyle and follow some exercise routine. When you combine all these, ayurvedic treatment does work. Many studies have shown that ayurvedic medicines bring down blood sugar. But what you need to remember is that ayurvedic treatment may not fully normalize your blood sugar. So after trying ayurvedic treatment, if your blood sugar is still not under control, do not go on for years hoping that blood sugar will come down one day. Because, if your blood sugar remains high for many years, you may develop blood vessel blocks, kidney, eye, and nerve damage. There is no harm if you want to try ayurvedic medicines or continue them along with modern medicines.

Homeopathy

Homeopathy says that if a substance produces any disease, the same substance taken in very minute quantities can cure that disease. Effectiveness of homeopathy in curing or controlling diabetes is yet to be proven. So do not skip your usual diabetes medicines or insulin while trying homeopathic medicines. You can try homeopathic medicines for sometime if your blood sugar is not dangerously high. Then be quick to consult a doctor who practices modern medicine if your blood sugar is not controlled within a few months.

Yoga and Pranayama

Yoga and pranayama can help you in many ways. It can help you in controlling blood sugars, manage stress more effectively, and contribute to overall health. Full benefits of yoga cannot be explained scientifically, though everyone who practices it can feel the good effects within a few months. It is a very good idea to include some yoga and pranayama in your daily routine. But do not stop your diabetes medicines and continue only yoga and pranayama. Continue your medicines, and if yoga and pranayama brings down blood sugar, you should be able to reduce the dose of medicines. If you require same dose of medicines as it was before starting yoga and pranayama, it means yoga is not having any effect on your blood sugar.

Acupuncture

In acupuncture, small needles are inserted into the skin to manipulate energy flow through invisible channels. Acupuncture believes that there are numerous energy channels in the body which are invisible. It is like electromagnetic flow. Diseases are produced due to either excess flow of energy or decreased flow of energy. Needles are inserted into these channels either to increase or decrease energy and thereby cure or control a disease. Do not mistake these energy channels for blood vessels or nerves. They are different from blood vessels and nerves. Though the existence of these channels is not proven by science, you need not rely on science to prove everything. Science has limitations and there are many things, which are true but cannot be explained by science. Some Western scientists believe that acupuncture triggers the release of the body's natural painkillers. Acupuncture has been shown to offer relief from chronic pain. Acupuncture is sometimes used by people with diabetic neuropathy to control pain.

A FINAL ADVICE

Every medical science has advantages and disadvantages. You can make the best use of everything. Perhaps it is best to use modern medicines to keep blood sugar under control, do some yoga and pranayama to reduce stress and tone up your body and mind, live an ayurvedic lifestyle to prevent diseases and improve health. But always keep your eye on the blood sugar levels. Do not continue any alternative medical therapy that is not controlling your blood sugar within a reasonable time (may be a few months if blood sugar is not very high). It is foolish to continue such medicines for many years and leave your blood sugar uncontrolled. Because, once you develop damage to your eyes, kidneys, blood vessels and heart, they may not be fully reversible. It is also foolish to try such therapies without modern medicines when your blood sugar is very high, say more than 300 mg/dl.

19 Visiting Your Doctor

Being a diabetic, you need to keep in touch with your doctor frequently. You should take an active role in your health care, which can help you get the best care possible from your doctor.

Tips to get the best out of your visit with your doctor

- Tell your doctor all about your complaints and illnesses whether current or past problem. It is better to note down your complaints in a notebook and bring it with you; otherwise, you may forget to tell some information. Take care not to waste your doctor's time. For example, do not go on telling how much runs you used to make during school cricket or how many medals you won. Do not get embarrassed to share any personal information like sexual contacts, drinking, and smoking.
- Tell your doctor about any medicines you are currently taking. Bring the old prescriptions and if possible medicines themselves. You should note down the strength of your tablets (e.g. Daonil 2.5 mg or 5 mg?) and how many times you are taking them. Also bring the insulin bottle or pen with you. Tell your doctor about any side effects you are experiencing. Always tell your doctor about any medicine to which you are allergic. If you are taking any vitamins or supplements with or without prescription tell your doctor about them also.
- Bring along with you any x-rays, scans, tests results or medical records you have and show them to your doctor. It is better to maintain a diary of your blood sugar tests, BP and weight recordings so that your doctor can assess the trend.
- Don't be afraid to ask questions. Ask your doctor about anything which you do not understand. Many people have doubts about whether to take a medicine before or after meals, how many times to take etc. clarify all these if you don't understand.

- It is good idea to write down any information or instructions that your doctor tells you so that you will not forget them later. Sometimes it helps to bring a friend or family member with you. They can help you remember the instructions or write it down for you.
- Do not feel embarrassed to contact the nurse, doctor's assistant or doctor if you are confused about something after you come back from visit.

How frequently should you visit your doctor?

If you are a newly diagnosed diabetic, initially it may be necessary to visit your doctor once a week to adjust medicines or insulin.

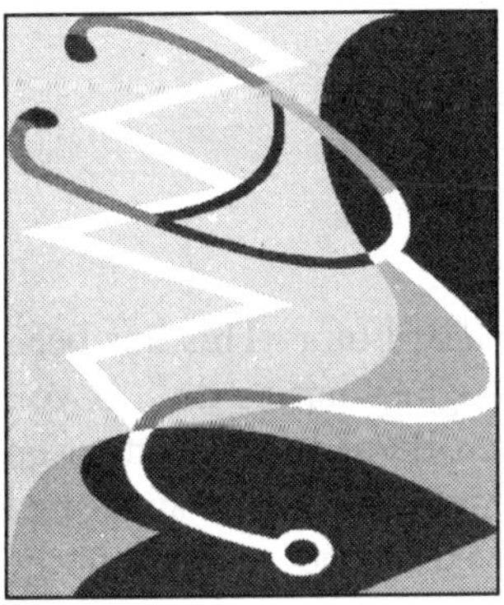

If your blood sugar is very high or you have some complication like DKA, you may require admission for a few days. Once your blood sugars are controlled and stable then your visits can be less frequent. Any way let your doctor decide how frequently you have to visit him. Periodic check ups are important to control your diabetes effectively and prevent long-term complications associated with diabetes.

In addition to this, you need to consult an eye specialist once a year and get your eyes checked for any early signs of retinopathy. Early diagnosis means easy treatment and better chances of cure. Your physician will usually refer you for eye check ups. If not remind him about this.

Emergency Visits

Consult your doctor immediately or go to any well-equipped hospital if you experience any of the following:

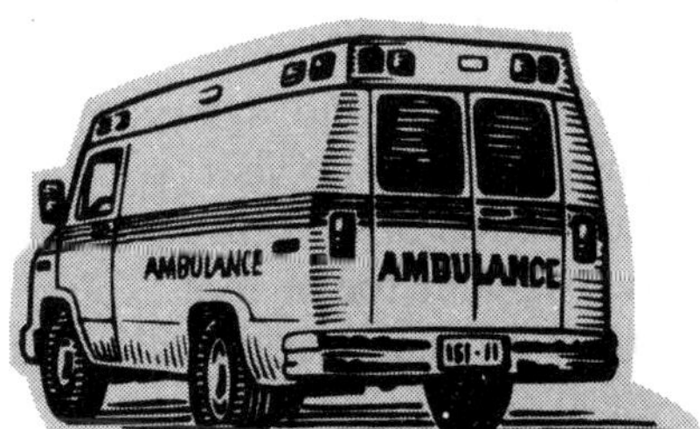

Symptoms of DKA and HHS

- Increased thirst and urination
- Nausea or/and vomiting

- Deep and fast breathing
- Abdominal pain
- Sweet-smelling breath
- Drowsiness or unconsciousness

Symptoms of hypoglycemia

- Trembling
- Weakness
- Drowsiness
- Headache
- Confusion
- Dizziness
- Double vision
- Speech problem
- Convulsions or unconsciousness

You can treat hypoglycemia yourself at home. This has been explained in the chapter "low blood sugar-what to do". If you can correct hypoglycemia yourself then there is no need to go to hospital. However, if the hypoglycemia is severe as suggested by fits, unconsciousness then you need to be rushed to the hospital immediately.

Signs of infection or gangrene.

- High grade fever, severe weakness,
- Cough and breathlessness
- Swollen and red leg or infection anywhere
- Blackish discoloration of toes

These signs and symptoms suggest serious infection and should make you visit your doctor immediately. Blackish discoloration of toes suggests onset of gangrene. If delayed you may lose your toe or foot. You may require hospital admission to treat all these serious illnesses.

20 Common Myths about Diabetes

Right knowledge is a boon and wrong knowledge a bane. Ignorance is better than having wrong knowledge. There are some misconceptions about diabetes, which have developed over the years. It is important to be aware of these so that you do not have unnecessary fears about them.

Myth 1. Diabetes is a serious illness and people with diabetes cannot lead a normal life

No, not at all. It is a serious mistake to believe this. Almost all people with diabetes can live a normal life. If you follow a healthy lifestyle and keep your blood sugar under control, then diabetes is not a serious illness at all.

Myth 2. Eating sweets and sugar causes diabetes

This is a common belief among people. The truth is that eating sweets and sugar does not cause diabetes. However, it may make a person overweight, which is a risk factor for developing diabetes. If you are already a diabetic, you need to cut down on sweets to keep your blood sugar under good control.

Myth 3. A person with diabetes should not eat fruits, because fruits contain sugar

You can eat fruits but within limits. One fruit per day does not harm you and does lot of good things to you like providing vitamins and minerals. What you should be careful is your total calories should not go high. You can eat fruit but cut down something else to keep the total calories same as recommended (e.g. reduce the quantity of rice or cut down one chapatti). A dietician can construct a diet chart that includes some fruits daily and at the same time keeping your total calories as required.

Myth 4. Stress causes diabetes

It does not cause diabetes. It does not have any direct relation to diabetes. However, if a person already has diabetes stress can make it worse.

Myth 5. Diabetes spreads from one person to another

The truth is that it does not. It is not contagious. Someone with diabetes cannot pass it on to anyone else. However, if a close relative has diabetes, then other family members have more chances of developing it. This is not because of close contact but because of genetic predisposition. There may be some genes, which make a person more prone to develop diabetes, and these genes may be transmitted genetically.

Myth 6. If you take insulin once, then you should always take it

No, not always. Many times doctors may put you on insulin only temporarily. For example, if your blood sugar is very high, if you are undergoing some surgery, or if you have some illness. Once these problems are settled, you can be put back on tablets. There are situations like type 1 diabetes and advanced stages of type 2 diabetes where you need to take insulin on a permanent basis.

Myth 7. Diabetes can be cured by other systems of medicine like ayurveda, herbal medicine, homeopathy etc.

So far, there is no proof that any system of medicine cures diabetes. Diabetes can only be kept under control. Sometimes initial stages of diabetes can be cured by proper diet, healthy lifestyle, and weight reduction. One should not believe any tall claims without scientific proof as this may lead to unnecessary trial of ineffective medicines and uncontrolled blood sugars.

Myth 8. Diabetics should not eat rice

Rice and chapattis are similar and contain almost similar amounts of carbohydrates. Rice can be eaten by all means.

Myth 9. Honey is good for diabetes

Honey contains lots of sugar and is rich in calories. Taking large quantity can push blood sugar out of control.

Myth 10. Extra diabetes pill before or after eating a large meal or sweet will control blood sugar

Many patients take an extra half to one tablet with, before or after a large meal hoping that, it will cover the extra large meal or sweet. Though insulin can be increased by 1 or 2 units before a large meal or feast, taking extra tablets is not advisable as tablets are not designed to cover 1 meal. Most of them act for full day, which may lead to erratic sugar control with swings of high and low blood sugar.

21 Is there a Permanent Cure for Diabetes?

This is the dream of every diabetic and the goal of many scientists. Research is going on to find a way to cure diabetes permanently and some of them have met with some success. The following is a small introduction to what is happening around the world.

Before I introduce you towards some research, which is going on to find permanent cure for diabetes, let me tell you that you yourself can cure your diabetes if it is type 2 diabetes, and is in early stage. It is possible by adopting healthy life style. By healthy lifestyle, I mean, eat healthy food (lots of vegetables, less of fats and oils, less of non-veg), exercise regularly, do some yoga and pranayama, reduce your weight if you are overweight, quit bad habits like smoking and drinking alcohol. Many diabetics are able to stop tablets by adopting healthy lifestyle and maintaining normal body weight. For people with type 1 diabetes and advanced type 2 diabetes there is hope of permanent cure by pancreas transplantation and islet cell transplantation.

Pancreas transplantation

Pancreas transplants have been performed since the late 1960s. We know that in diabetics the beta cells in pancreas are not working properly. Therefore, if we can change the pancreas then potentially diabetes can be cured. But there are many problems with pancreas transplantation. First thing is, pancreas is difficult to get like kidney. Second is your body may reject any new organ which is put into you from somebody else. So you need to get pancreas from a matching donor. Even then, your body may not accept an organ from somebody else. To make the body accept the organ, you need to take some medicines, which will cost you any where between Rs.5000 to 15,000 and you need to take these medicines lifelong. These drugs have serious side effects, including high risk of infection and organ injury. Because the side effects can be more dangerous to your health than your diabetes, you are usually not considered a candidate for transplantation unless your diabetes cannot be controlled or you are experiencing serious complications.

Islet cell transplantation

We know that insulin comes from beta cells of pancreas. These beta cells are present in groups, which are called as islet cells. Therefore, what about transplanting islet cells instead of whole of pancreas? This seems to be a good idea although still considered an experimental procedure. Transplanting islet cells is less expensive and less risky than a pancreas transplant. In islet cell transplantation, doctors infuse fresh islet cells into the liver of the person with diabetes. The cells spread throughout the liver and soon begin to produce insulin. Islets can also be transplanted into forearm.

There is definitely a chance for curing diabetes permanently if the ongoing research succeeds. However, you need to wait for some more time until all the doubts about these procedures are cleared.

22 Eleven Things you should Always Follow

In life, there are no shortcuts. If you want to be successful, you need to follow some discipline and managing diabetes is no different. Follow the ten things given below and you will be surprised about how healthy you will be.

1. Visit your doctor at least 4 times a year or more times if required.
2. Check your blood sugar regularly and get your medicines or insulin adjusted by your doctor. Take your medicines regularly. This will keep your blood sugar always under control.
3. Check your BP regularly at least once in 3 months if under control and more frequently if not under control. Keeping your BP within normal range is vital to prevent complications. Take your BP medicines regularly if any.
4. Get your glycosylated hemoglobin (HbA1c) tested once in 3 months. This will show you whether your blood sugar is in good control or not.
5. Get your cholesterol levels checked every year and if high get necessary treatment for this.
6. Get your eyes checked at least once a year. By doing this, you can prevent permanent eye damage and blindness.
7. Get dental check and cleaning every 6 months. Inform dentist that you have diabetes.
8. Check your feet every day for signs of injury or infection. Take care of your feet the way you take care of your face.
9. Do some regular exercise. Exercise not only controls your diabetes, but also improves your overall health.
10. Stick to the correct diet recommended to you.
11. Always carry with you some identification, which mentions that you are a diabetic. Also, carry some chocolates, sweets, or sugar cubes with you. It will help in emergencies.

23 Diabetes Dictionary

You may come across many medical words when you are reading newspapers, listening to a TV interview or talking to your doctor. Some of the most commonly used medical words and what they mean are given below.

Albumin

Albumin is a protein present in blood. It normally does not leak into the urine. When kidney is damaged, it leaks into the urine. Hence, presence of albumin in the urine usually suggests kidney damage.

Amino Acids

These are the building blocks of proteins. Many amino acids combine to make a protein. Insulin is also a protein and made of 51 amino acids. Amino acids are essential for our body and we obtain them from food.

Angina

Angina is left sided chest pain that is due to decreased blood supply to heart. It becomes more on exertion and decreases on resting. If angina is very severe, it can lead to heart attack.

Antibodies

Antibodies are proteins, which act against something and inactivate or destroy it. It may be virus, bacteria, or our own tissues. In type 1 diabetes, there are antibodies against beta cells of pancreas, which destroy them.

Atherosclerosis

This is nothing but collection of cholesterol and fibrous tissue inside blood vessels. The result is blocking of blood vessels, which can lead to heart attack, stroke, or gangrene of toes.

Autoimmunity

Auto means self. Autoimmunity means immunity against ones own tissues due to antibodies. Example is antibodies against beta cells of pancreas. Normally we do not have antibodies, which react against our own body.

Beta Cells

Beta cells are special cells present in pancreas. They produce insulin. Destruction of beta cells leads to less production of insulin, which in turn leads to diabetes.

Blood pressure

This is the pressure inside blood vessels. It is not mental tension as mistaken by many people. High blood pressure can lead to blocks or rupture of blood vessels. High blood pressure also causes heart attacks, stroke, and kidney damage.

Cataract

There is a lens in our eye, which is transparent like glass. We see the world through this transparent lens. Formation of opacities in the lens is called cataract, because of which we cannot see properly and our eyesight becomes blurred. Treatment for this is cataract surgery where the opacities are removed from the lens or the whole lens is removed and a new artificial lens is put.

Cholesterol

This is a type of fat in the body. There is good cholesterol (HDL-cholesterol) and bad cholesterol (LDL-cholesterol) in the body. You should have more of good and less of bad cholesterol in the body. Cholesterol gets collected inside blood vessels and blocks them causing heart attack, stroke, and kidney damage. There are medicines to decrease cholesterol level called statins.

Coma

Coma is complete loss of consciousness. Patient appears as if he is sleeping but cannot be woken up. There are many reasons for it and it can happen in severe hypoglycemia, DKA, and HHS.

Creatinine

Creatinine is a waste product produced in the body. It is filtered by the kidney and thrown out in the urine. When there is kidney damage creatinine levels in the blood start rising. So high blood creatinine levels indicate significant kidney damage.

Dawn Phenomenon

In early morning time, many hormones like growth hormone, cortisol are secreted more. This is a natural phenomenon. These hormones cause increase in blood sugar early in the morning, which is known as dawn phenomenon.

Dialysis

Dialysis is a method to clean the blood when kidneys have failed. Normally kidneys filter the blood and remove waste products. Dialysis machine does the same when kidneys have failed.

Diabetes insipidus

Do not mistake this for diabetes mellitus. Diabetes insipidus is a disease where large amount of urine is passed. It is due to some defect in the brain or kidneys. Blood sugars are normal in this disease.

Diabetic neuropathy

Uncontrolled diabetes can damage nerves in the body, which is known as diabetic neuropathy. Symptoms include tingling, numbness and burning in the feet initially. Later this happens in the hands also.

Diabetic nephropathy

Uncontrolled diabetes damages kidneys. Initially this is known by presence of albumin in the urine. Later on there is rise of urea and creatinine in the blood. In the last stages, dialysis may be required.

Diabetic retinopathy

This is damage to retina due to diabetes. Retina is a light sensitive structure made of small nerves inside the eye. Without this we cannot see. In diabetes, blood vessels supplying retina get blocked and cause damage to retina which is known as diabetic retinopathy. Retinopathy can be prevented by good sugar control. Test your eyes every year to detect early diabetic retinopathy.

Diabetic foot

Diabetics often have foot problems. It may be ulcers, infection, or gangrene. All these are called diabetic foot.

Dietary Fiber

This is present in veg food. It cannot be digested by us. However, it does many good things for us. It prevents constipation. It prevents intestinal cancer. It reduces your weight. So include more vegetables in your diet

FBS (Fasting blood sugar)

This is the blood sugar test done in the morning without taking any food. Dinner can be taken but after dinner, no food should be taken except water. A value more than 126 mg/dl indicates diabetes.

Gestational Diabetes

This is diabetes, which comes only during pregnancy. Most of the oral medicines cannot be used and it requires insulin throughout pregnancy. If uncontrolled, it can harm both the mother and the baby.

Glucagon

This is a hormone produced by pancreas. It has effects exactly opposite to insulin. It helps in correcting low blood sugar as happens in fasting or after taking excess dose of insulin. Glucagon injections are available and you should keep one at home. In emergencies when blood sugar becomes low, you or your family members can inject it to you.

Glycogen

Glycogen is a storage form of glucose. When glucose is high, some of it is converted into glycogen and stored in liver and muscles. When glucose becomes low, glycogen can again be converted into glucose.

HbA1c

This is hemoglobin, which has combined with glucose. Higher the glucose, higher the HbA1c value. It gives an idea about blood sugar control over the last 3 months. Normally it should be less than 7%. If more than this, it indicates poor sugar control. Check your HbA1c once in 3 months.

Hyperglycemia

It is just another name for high blood sugar.

Hyperlipidemia

This is a general term for increased fats (lipids) in the blood. These fats may be triglycerides, cholesterol etc. Hyperlipidemia leads to blood vessel blocks and needs to be treated.

Hypoglycemia

This is just another name for low blood sugar. If blood sugar is less than 60 mg/dl, it is called hypoglycemia.

Hypoglycemia Unawareness

Normally a person can recognize hypoglycemia by symptoms like sweating, shaking, weakness etc. Sometimes these symptoms may be absent, and the person cannot recognize hypoglycemia. This is called hypoglycemia unawareness. It can happen in advanced stages of diabetes due to nerve damage.

Injection Site Rotation

Changing the injection site daily is called Injection Site Rotation. It is not that one day you inject into abdomen and another day into arms etc. It means you inject into same area but change the position daily. Injection site rotation prevents local skin damage.

Insulin

This is a protein hormone secreted by beta cells of pancreas. Its main job is to make the body use glucose. When insulin is less or absent in the body it leads to high blood sugars which is known as diabetes mellitus.

Insulin Pump

This is a small instrument, which is worn on the body, and it pumps insulin continuously into the body. There is no need to inject insulin manually once it is fixed. They are not widely used but very useful for some.

Insulin Resistance

A person with insulin resistance does not react normally to insulin as a normal person does. Hence, even if insulin levels are normal blood sugar becomes high. This happens in type 2 diabetes.

Ketones

These are produced by the body when fat is burnt to produce energy rather than glucose. Sometimes this happens in diabetic who is not able to use glucose due to lack of insulin. Presence of ketones in the urine should be taken seriously because it may lead to DKA.

Lactic Acidosis

This is collection of lactic acid in the body. It is a serious condition. It can happen in people taking metformin especially if they have kidney damage.

Lancet

This is a small sharp object used to puncture fingertip to obtain a drop of blood. This blood drop is put on glucose strip inserted into a glucometer, which measures sugar level.

Lipid Profile

Lipid profile is a blood test which measures the levels of all fats like cholesterol, triglycerides etc. It is usually done in the morning on empty stomach, hence also called fasting lipid profile. A person with diabetes needs to test his lipid profile periodically.

Microalbuminuria

Presence of albumin in micro quantities in the urine is called microalbuminuria. It indicates early kidney damage.

Myocardial infraction

This is the medical word for heart attack. Here blood vessels supplying heart suddenly get blocked which leads to death of heart muscle. This is known as heart attack. This is a serious condition and a medical emergency. When it happens, the person experiences severe left sided chest pain. Sometimes the pain is felt in the upper abdomen and is mistaken for gas or gastritis. If you are a diabetic beware of any gas or gastritis, it may be heart attack. Consult your doctor immediately.

Nocturnal Hypoglycemia

This is low blood sugar happening at night when you may be sleeping. It may go unnoticed because of sleep. It is important to prevent this by having some bedtime snacks and correctly adjusting your tablets and insulin. Never skip your dinner.

Ophthalmologist

A doctor who specializes in eye diseases. You need to meet him at least once a year to get your eyes checked. Your family doctor or physician will usually refer you to him.

Oral Glucose Tolerance Test (OGTT)

This is the ideal test to diagnose whether one has diabetes but usually not necessary.

Pancreas

A organ present in the abdomen. It secretes many enzymes, which digest our food. Beta cells, which secrete insulin, are also present in pancreas. Glucogon is also secreted from pancreas.

Pancreatitis

This is a disease of pancreas where there is infection or inflammation. Bleeding and pus formation can occur inside pancreas. Pancreas stops producing insulin and the person may develop diabetes. Most of the time tablets will not work for this type of diabetes, and hence insulin has to be given.

Peripheral Vascular Disease (PVD)

This is a disease of blood vessels of legs and arms. Blood vessels get blocked either partially or completely which lead to pain in the legs while walking or gangrene. There is also a risk of developing ulcers because of decreased blood supply. Reasons for PVD are many like diabetes, hypertension etc.

PPBS (Postprandial blood sugar)

This is blood sugar measurement done usually 2 hours after eating. It can be done after breakfast, after lunch or after dinner. It should not go more than 140 mg/dl in a normal person.

Prediabetes

A stage where you neither have normal blood sugar to call you as normal nor have high blood sugar to call you as a diabetic. It is the early stage of diabetes. When you have this, you need to be careful and do some exercise and eat healthy food to prevent progression to frank diabetes.

Pressure Sore

This is a wound, which develops on the pressure areas like soles of your feet. It happens because you may have decreased sensation in the feet due to nerve damage (diabetic neuropathy). Hence, small injuries on pressure points go unnoticed and develop into sores.

Proteinuria

This is presence of proteins in urine. It happens in kidney damage because proteins from blood start leaking into urine. Albuminuria is the commonest proteinuria.

RBS (Random blood sugar)

This is blood sugar test done at any time of the day without bothering about the time of food intake. A value more than 200 mg/dl suggests diabetes.

Stroke

This is sudden onset of weakness, speaking difficulty or unconsciousness. Most common type is weakness of one side of the body. This is either due to blockage of blood vessels in the brain or due to rupture of damaged blood vessels. Diabetics have more chance of having a stroke especially if the sugar remains uncontrolled.

APPENDIX- I

FOOD GROUPS AND EXCHANGES

Our food items can be grouped into 8 groups. You can choose food items from each group or choose more items in one group. Once you know how many calories you should take per day, choose the appropriate diet chart from appendix-III. Suppose you have chosen 1500-calorie veg diet chart, in that chart for breakfast you have the option of 2 cereal exchanges. Now, you can choose 2 cereal exchanges in the cereal group table. E.g., you can choose 1 large slice bread and 1 chapatti. Similarly, in the same diet chart, it is written ½ milk exchange for morning tea. For this, you can choose ½-cup whole milk or 4 ounz plain whole yogurt. Note that in diet charts, 3 cereal means 3 cereal exchanges. Similarly, 3 milk means 3 milk exchanges and not 3 cups of milk.

Cereal Group

The cereal group forms the large portion of your meal. Each serving of cereal shown below gives about 80 calories.

Cereal Group

Food Item	*Quantity which Provides 80 Calories*
Wheat Flour, Ragi Flour, Bajra Flour, Kotu Flour, Maida	25 gms
Bread (White or Brown)	1 large slice, or two small slices or 25 gms
Chapattis (Wheat, Jowar, Bajra or Maize)	1 Chapatti, approx. 6 inches wide or 25 gms weight
Dalia Cooked	½ cup

Dosa	1, approx. 10 inches in diameter or 40 gms weight
Idli	1 small approx. 30 gms. weight
Macaroni cooked	½ cup
Noodles cooked	½ cup
Pau	1 average size
Poha	½ cup
Porridge	½ cup
Potato	1 small, 2½ in. diameter
Raw Plantain	½ cup
Rice, white or brown, boiled	½ cup
Rice, flaked	25 gms weight
Spaghetti cooked	½ cup
Sweet Potato (shakarkhandi)	1/3rd cup
Upma	½ cup
Yam (Suran)	1/3rd cup

Vegetables Group

Vegetables are not rich in calories, but provide lots of vitamins and minerals. Each vegetable serving shown below gives approximately 28 calories.

Vegetables Group

Food Item	*Quantity which Provides 28 Calories*
Amaranth (Chola)	½ cup cooked
Ash gourd (Petha)	½ cup cooked
Asparagus	½ cup cooked
Bananas raw	½ cup cooked
Bean sprouts	½ cup cooked
Beans	½ cup cooked
Beetroot	½ cup cooked
Beets	½ cup cooked
Bhindi (Ladies Fingers)	½ cup cooked

Bitter gourd (Karela)	½ cup cooked
Bottle gourd (Lauki)	½ cup cooked
Brinjal (Baingan)	½ cup cooked
Broad beans (Papadi)	½ cup cooked
Broccoli	½ cup cooked
Brussels sprouts	½ cup cooked
Cabbage, cooked	½ cup cooked
Capsicum (Shimla Mirch)	½ cup cooked
Carrots	½ cup cooked or 1 cup raw
Cauliflower	½ cup cooked
Cauliflower (Phool Gobi)	½ cup cooked
Cluster beans (Gawar)	½ cup cooked
Drumsticks (Saijan Ki Phalli)	½ cup cooked
French beans (Fansi)	½ cup cooked
Gourd ash (Petha)	½ cup cooked
Greens (Collard, Mustard, Turnip)	½ cup cooked
Cucumber	½ cup cooked or 1 cup raw
Khol Khol (Ganth Gobi)	½ cup cooked
Methi (Fenugreek)	½ cup cooked
Mushrooms, Cooked	½ cup cooked
Onions	½ cup cooked or 1 cup raw
Parva, (Ordinary)	½ cup cooked
Parval (Long)	½ cup cooked
Pea pods	½ cup cooked
Peas (Mutter)	½ cup cooked
Peppers (green)	½ cup cooked
Pumpkin	½ cup cooked
Radish (muli)	½ cup cooked or 1 cup raw
Ridge gourd (turiya)	½ cup cooked
Rutabaga	½ cup cooked
Salad mixed	1 cup
Spinach	½ cup cooked or 1 cup raw
Summer squash (crookneck)	½ cup cooked or 1 cup raw
Tomato/tomato juice	one large or ½ cup juice
Vegetable juice	Three/quarters cup
Turnips	½ cup cooked

Pulses and Dals

Pulses and dals are rich in proteins and carbohydrates. They contain more protein than cereal group. Each serving in this group as shown below gives approximately 80 calories.

Pulses and Dals Group

Food Item	*Quantity which Provides 80 Calories*
Dal, Masoor	25 gms (if uncooked), 1 cup (if cooked, thin and watery), ½ cup (if cooked and thick)
Dal, Arhar	Same as above
Dal, Urad	Same as above
Dal, Tur (Red Gram)	Same as above
Dal, Mooth (Mothbeans)	Same as above
Val (Field Beans)	Same as above
Moong (Greengram)	Same as above
Peas Dry	Same as above
Rajmah	Same as above
Chana (Bengal Gram)	Same as above
Kidney Beans	Same as above
Lentils	Same as above
Beans	1/3 cup
Peas, Cooked	1/3 cup
Kidney Beans, Cooked.	1/3 cup
Lentils, Cooked	1/3 cup
Red beans, Cooked.	1/3 cup

Milk and Milk Products

Milk and milk products are rich in proteins, calcium, vitamins and minerals. Each serving in this group as shown below gives approximately 80 calories.

Milk and Milk Products

Food Item	*Quantity which Provides 80 Calories*
Skim milk	1 cup
Low-fat or nonfat buttermilk	1 cup
Flavored Yogurt without sugar	1 cup
Plain nonfat yogurt	¾ cup
Any cottage cheese	1/3 cup
Diet cheese (with less than 55 calories per ounce)	One and half ounce
All other cheeses	1 oz (30 gms)
Whole milk	1 cup
Evaporated whole milk	½ cup
Whole plain yogurt	8 oz
Goat's milk	1 cup
Kefir	1 cup

Fruits

Fruits are rich in vitamins and minerals. Since fruits are sweet and contain sugar, they should be eaten in restricted quantities. Each serving in this group as shown below gives approximately 60 calories.

Fruits

Fruits	*Quantity which Provides 60 Calories*
Apple	1, two inch wide
Amla (Indian Gooseberry)	15
Anjir (Figs)	2, large size
Apple Juice/Cider	½ cup
Apricots, Raw	4
Avocado	2, medium
Banana (9″ Long)	1/2 banana
Blackberries (raw)	¾ cup
Blueberries (raw)	¾ cup
Cantaloupe Melon	¼, medium size

Cherries	12, large size
Cherries (Canned)	½ cup
Chikoo	1, small
Cranberry Juice Cocktail	1/3 cup
Dates (fresh)	3, medium size
Figs (raw, 2" across)	2 figs
Galia melon	¼, medium size
Grape juice	1/3 cup
Grapefruit (medium)	½ grapefruit, 3½ inch wide, ¾ cup pieces or ½ cup juice
Grapes	15, small size
Guava	1, medium size
Jackfruit	3, medium size
Jambu (white)	15 pieces
Kiwi (Large)	1 Kiwi
Mango	½ small
Melon (honeydew)	¼ medium size
Muskmelon (musk)	¼ medium size
Orange	1 orange (2½" across) or ½ cup juice
Papaya	1 cup
Peaches	1, 2 ½ wide
Peaches (canned)	½ cup or 2 halves
Pear	½ large, or 1 small
Pineapple (canned)	½ cup
Pineapple (raw)	¾ cup
Pineapple juice	½ cup
Pomegranate	½ pomegranate
Prunes	3 medium or 1/3 cup juice
Raisins	2 tbsp.
Raspberries	1 cup
Seetaphal	½, medium size
Strawberries	1¼ cup
Sweet lime	1, 2½ wide
Tangerine (2½" across)	2 tangerines
Watermelon (cubed)	1¼ cup

Fats and Oils

Fats and oils are rich in cholesterol and calories. They make the food tastier. They should be used sparingly. Each serving as shown below gives 45 calories.

Fats and Oils

Food Item	*Quantity which Provides 45 Calories*
Cooking oil	1 tablespoon
Salad dressing	1 tablespoon
Margarine	1 teaspoon
Mayonnaise	1 teaspoon
Ghee	1 teaspoon
Butter	1-1/4 teaspoon

Meats

Meats are rich in proteins and calories. Now-a-days veg foods are preferred over meats. Each meat serving shown below gives roughly 55 calories.

Meats

Food Item	*Quantity which Provides 55 Calories*
Poultry (Chicken, Turkey)	1 oz (30 gms)
Fish	1 oz (30 gms)
Crab, Lobster	2 oz (60 gms)
Oysters	6 medium
Beef	lean, without fat-1 oz medium fat- ¾ oz high fat- ½ oz
Pork	lean, without fat-1 oz medium fat- ¾ oz high fat- ½ oz
Lamb	lean, without fat-1 oz medium fat- ¾ oz high fat- ½ oz

Free Foods

Free foods provide less than 20 calories per serving. Hence, they can be taken little freely whenever you feel hungry.

Free Foods

Food Item	*Provide Less than 20 Calories per serving*
Cucumber	1 serving
Green onion	1 serving
Candy, hard, sugar-free	1
Carbonated water	1 serving
Club Soda	1 serving
Cocoa Powder, without Sugar	(1 tbsp.)
Coffee/Tea Sugar Free	1 cup
Gelatin, sugar-free	2 tsp
Jam/Jelly, sugar-free	2 tsp
Sugar substitutes (saccharin, aspartame)	2 tsp
Vinegar	2 tsp
Curry	1 serving
Flavoring extracts (Vanilla, Peppermint, Lemon, etc.)	1 serving
Hot pepper sauce	2 tsp
Lemon juice	1 glass
Mint	1 serving
Soya sauce	2 tsp
Soup, clear	1 cup
Tonic Water, Sugar-free	2 tsp

APPENDIX- II

DIET CHARTS

How to use diet charts?

The first step towards using diet charts is to know how many calories you should eat per day. You can know the number of calories required by you per day by referring to chart in chapter 5. You can also know this from your doctor or dietician. The charts given below are constructed to provide 1200, 1500, 1800, 2100, and 2400 calories. If your required number of calories is same as one of these charts, you can straight away use the charts. If your required number of calories is not same as one of these charts, you can modify these charts to make the required calories. For example, suppose your requirement is 1400 calories for which there is no chart here, you can remove food items worth 100 calories from 1500-calorie chart and make a 1400-calorie chart. This can be done by skipping 1 cereal exchange (equals 80 calories) and ½ fat exchange (roughly equals 20 calories) from 1500 calorie diet chart. Similarly, you can make charts for any required calories.

While using diet charts, note that the number in front of food groups indicates number of exchanges. Vegetable 2 does not mean 2 carrots or 2 beetroots. It means 2 vegetable exchanges, which is equal to 1-cup carrot or 1-cup beetroot as per the quantities shown in appendix-I. All the exchanges are given in appendix-I, which you can choose according to your wish. For example to choose 1 cereal exchange, you have many options if you refer to cereal group in appendix-I.

Also, note that in diet charts one of the milk exchanges per day is whole milk. For example in 1200-calorie diet, out of 2 milk exchanges allowed, one should be whole milk and other can be anything as per your choice (say buttermilk).

Vegetarian Diet—1200 CALORIES

Exchanges: 6 Cereal, 2 Milk, 5 Veg, 2 Fruits, 2 Pulses, 3 Fats/Oils

Morning Tea/Coffee	Milk ½				
Breakfast	Cereal 1½	Milk ½	Vegetable 1	Fat/oil 1	
Mid-Morning Snack	Free foods				
Lunch	Cereal 2	Milk ½	Vegetable 2	Pulses 1	Fat/oil 1
Evening Tea/coffee	Free food				
Dinner	Cereal 2½	Milk ½	Vegetable 2	Pulses 1	Fat/oil 1
Bedtime	Milk ½				

Vegetarian Diet—1500 CALORIES

Exchanges: 8 Cereal, 3 Milk, 5 Veg, 2 Fruits, 2 Pulses, 4 Fats/Oils

Morning Tea/Coffee	Milk ½				
Breakfast	Cereal 2	Milk 1	Vegetable 1	Fat/oil 1	
Mid-Morning Snack	Free food				
Lunch	Cereal 2	Milk ½	Vegetable 2	Pulses 1	Fat/oil 1½
Evening Tea/coffee	Cereal 1	Free food			
Dinner	Cereal 3	Milk ½	Vegetable 2	Pulses 1	Fat/oil 1½
Bedtime	Milk ½				

Vegetarian diet—1800 CALORIES

Exchanges: 10 Cereal, 4 Milk, 5 Veg, 2 Fruits, 3 Pulses, 4 Fats/Oils

Morning Tea/Coffee	Milk ½				
Breakfast	Cereal 2	Milk 1	Vegetable 1	Fat/oil 1	
Mid-Morning Snack	Free foods				
Lunch	Cereal 3	Milk 1	Vegetable 2	Pulses 2	Fat/oil 1½
Evening Tea/coffee	Cereal 1	Free foods	Milk ½		
Dinner	Cereal 4	Milk 1	Vegetable 2	Pulses 1½	Fat/oil 1½
Bedtime	Milk ½				

Vegetarian diet—2100 CALORIES

Exchanges: 12 Cereal, 4 Milk, 5 Veg, 3 Fruits, 3 Pulses, 5 Fats/Oils

Morning Tea/Coffee	Milk ½				
Breakfast	Cereal 3	Milk 1	Vegetable 1	Free foods	Fat/oil 1
Mid-Morning Snack	Free foods				
Lunch	Cereal 4	Milk 1	Vegetable 2	Pulses 1½	Fat/oil 2
Evening Tea/coffee	Cereal 1	Free foods			
Dinner	Cereal 4	Milk 1	Vegetable 2	Pulses 1½	Fat/oil 2
Bedtime	Milk ½				

Vegetarian diet—2400 CALORIES

Exchanges: 14 Cereal, 4 Milk, 5 Veg, 3 Fruits, 4 Pulses, 5 Fats/Oils

Morning Tea/Coffee	Milk ½				
Breakfast	Cereal 3	Milk 1	Vegetable 1	Free foods	Fat/oil 1
Mid-Morning Snack	Free foods				
Lunch	Cereal 4	Milk 1	Vegetable 2	Pulses 2	Fat/oil 2
Evening Tea/coffee	Cereal 2	Free foods			
Dinner	Cereal 5	Milk 1	Vegetable 2	Pulses 2	Fat/oil 2
Bedtime	Milk ½				

Non-Vegetarian diet—1200 CALORIES

Exchanges: 6 Cereal, 1½ Milk, 3 Vegetables, 3 Meat, 2 Fruits, 1½ Pulses, 3 Fats/Oils

Morning Tea/Coffee	Milk ½				
Breakfast	Cereal 1½	Milk ½	Meat 1	Fat/oil 1	
Mid-Morning Snack	Free foods				
Lunch	Cereal 2	Vegetable 1	Pulses 1	Meat 1	Fat/oil 1
Evening Tea/coffee	Free foods				
Dinner	Cereal 2½	Vegetable 2	Pulses ½	Meat 1	Fat/oil 1
Bedtime	Milk ½				

Non-Vegetarian diet—1500 CALORIES

Exchanges: 8 Cereal, 2½ Milk, 2 Vegetables, 4 Meat, 2 Fruits, 2 Pulses, 3 Fats/Oils

Morning Tea/Coffee	Milk ½					
Breakfast	Cereal 2	Milk ½	Meat 1	Fat/oil 1		
Mid-Morning Snack	Free foods					
Lunch	Cereal 2	Vegetable 1	Milk ½	Pulses 1	Meat 2	Fat/oil 1
Evening Tea/coffee	Free foods					
Dinner	Cereal 3	Vegetable 1	Pulses 1	Meat 1½	Fat/oil 1	
Bedtime	Milk ½					

Non-Vegetarian diet—1800 CALORIES

Exchanges: 10 Cereal, 2½ Milk, 3 Vegetables, 5 Meat, 2 Fruits, 2 Pulses, 4 Fats/Oils

Morning Tea/Coffee	Milk ½					
Breakfast	Cereal 2	Milk ½	Meat 1	Fat/oil 1		
Mid-Morning Snack	Free foods					
Lunch	Cereal 3	Vegetable 1	Milk ½	Meat 2	Pulses 1	Fat/oil 1½
Evening Tea/coffee	Cereal 1	Free foods	Milk ½			
Dinner	Cereal 4	Vegetable 2	Milk ½	Meat 2	Pulses 1	Fat/oil 1½
Bedtime	Milk ½					

Non-Vegetarian diet—2100 CALORIES

Exchanges: 12 Cereal, 3 Milk, 3 Vegetables, 5 Meat, 3 Fruits, 2 Pulses, 5 Fats/Oils

Morning Tea/Coffee	Milk ½					
Breakfast	Cereal 3	Milk ½	Meat 1	Free food	Fat/oil 1	
Mid-Morning Snack	Free food					
Lunch	Cereal 4	Vegetable 1	Milk ½	Meat 2	Pulses 1	Fat/oil 2
Evening Tea/coffee	Cereal 1	Free food	Milk ½			
Dinner	Cereal 4	Vegetable 2	Milk ½	Meat 2	Pulses 1	Fat/oil 2
Bedtime	Milk ½					

Non-Vegetarian diet—2400 CALORIES

Exchanges: 14 Cereal, 3 Milk, 3 Vegetables, 6 Meat, 3 Fruits, 2 Pulses, 6 Fats/Oils

Morning Tea/Coffee	Milk ½					
Breakfast	Cereal 3	Milk ½	Meat 1	Free foods	Fat/oil 2	
Mid-Morning Snack	Free foods					
Lunch	Cereal 5	Vegetable 1	Milk ½	Meat 2	Pulses 1	Fat/oil 2
Evening Tea/coffee	Cereal 2	Free foods	Milk ½			
Dinner	Cereal 4	Vegetable 2	Milk ½	Meat 3	Pulses 1	Fat/oil 2
Bedtime	Milk ½					

APPENDIX- III

DIABETES DIARY

It is important to write down your blood sugar reports, BP and weight recordings, hypoglycemia episodes, and HbA1c values in one place and keep it. Enter the results of your blood tests inside the respective boxes. Also, enter your weight and BP whenever you check it. Carry this diary with you, whenever you visit your doctor or hospital. It will be very easy for the doctor to go through the serial blood sugar results, assess control of sugar and BP to make necessary recommendations.

DATE									
FBS									
PPBS									
RBS									
BP									
CHOLESTEROL									
WEIGHT									

DATE									
HbA1c									

DATE and TIME									
Hypoglycemia (value)									

DATE									
FBS									
PPBS									
RBS									
BP									
CHOLESTEROL									
WEIGHT									

DATE									
HbA1c									

DATE and TIME									
Hypoglycemia (value)									

DATE									
FBS									
PPBS									
RBS									
BP									
CHOLESTEROL									
WEIGHT									

DATE									
HbA1c									

DATE and TIME									
Hypoglycemia (value)									

DATE									
FBS									
PPBS									
RBS									
BP									
CHOLESTEROL									
WEIGHT									

DATE									
HbA1c									

DATE and TIME									
Hypoglycemia (value)									

DATE									
FBS									
PPBS									
RBS									
BP									
CHOLESTEROL									
WEIGHT									

DATE									
HbA1c									

DATE and TIME									
Hypoglycemia (value)									

DATE									
FBS									
PPBS									
RBS									
BP									
CHOLESTEROL									
WEIGHT									

DATE									
HbA1c									

DATE and TIME									
Hypoglycemia (value)									

IMPORTANT PHONE NUMBERS

	Landline	*Mobile*
Ambulance		
Doctor (Family doctor)		
Doctor (physician)		
Nurse		
Diabetes educator		
Medical store		
Laboratory		
Friend		
Taxi		
Police		